Jane Bruce

Change Your Mood with Aromatherapy

D0610732

Teach
Yourself®

Change Your Mood with Aromatherapy

Denise Whichello Brown, BSc.,
Cert. Ed., DO, MIFPA, MIFR

Long renowned as the authoritative source for self-guided learning –
with more than 50 million copies sold worldwide – the **Teach Yourself**
series includes over 500 titles in the fields of languages, crafts, hobbies,
business, computing and education.

British Library Cataloguing in Publication Data: a catalogue record
for this title is available from the British Library.

Library of Congress Catalog Card Number: on file.

First published in UK 1996 by Hodder Education, part of
Hachette UK

First published in US 1996 by The McGraw-Hill Companies, Inc.

This edition published 2010.

Previously published as *Teach Yourself Aromatherapy*.

The **Teach Yourself** name is a registered trade mark of Hodder
Headline.

Copyright © 1996, 2001, 2003, 2007, 2010
Denise Whichello Brown

In UK: All rights reserved. Apart from any permitted use under UK
copyright law, no part of this publication may be reproduced or
transmitted in any form or by any means, electronic or mechanical,
including photocopy, recording, or any information, storage and
retrieval system, without permission in writing from the publisher
or under licence from the Copyright Licensing Agency Limited.
Further details of such licences (for reprographic reproduction)
may be obtained from the Copyright Licensing Agency Limited, of
Saffron House, 6–10 Kirby Street, London EC1N 8TS.

In US: All rights reserved. Except as permitted under the United
States Copyright Act of 1976, no part of this publication may
be reproduced or distributed in any form or by any means, or
stored in a database or retrieval system, without the prior written
permission of the publisher.

Typeset by MPS Limited, A Macmillan Company.

Printed in Great Britain for Hodder Education, an Hachette UK
Company

The publisher has used its best endeavours to ensure that the URLs
for external websites referred to in this book are correct and active
at the time of going to press. However, the publisher and the
author have no responsibility for the websites and can make no
guarantee that a site will remain live or that the content will remain
relevant, decent or appropriate.

Hachette UK's policy is to use papers that are natural, renewable
and recyclable products and made from wood grown in sustainable
forests. The logging and manufacturing processes are expected to
conform to the environmental regulations of the country of origin.

Year   2014 2013 2012 2011 2010

In loving memory of my dear friend Peter Grant, a true believer in the art of aromatherapy, who passed away shortly before the completion of this book.

Foreword

The way to health is to have an aromatic bath and scented massage every day.

Hippocrates

Hippocrates, the revered 'Father of Medicine', had great insight into the therapeutic value of many natural approaches to healing used in ancient Greece, including aromatherapy.

It seems paradoxical that, until recently, prior to commencing clinical practice in orthodox Western medicine, a universal requirement for the practising doctor was to take the 'Hippocratic Oath'. Yet, also until recently, aromatherapy, which was extolled by Hippocrates for its healing benefits, has been regarded with scepticism by the medical establishment regarding its therapeutic benefits. It has been considered to be simply a pleasant alternative therapy useful for soothing fraught nerves.

There is no doubt that calming the mind and relieving stress is of paramount importance in any healing process. However, aromatherapy offers much more. Over 300 aromatic oils are used by professional aromatherapists, although about ten would probably meet the everyday needs of the average family. Each oil has its own range of therapeutic properties dependent on the proportions and combinations of naturally occurring chemicals in the oil. Chemists have isolated 'active' ingredients from some of the oils which have shown by practical usage to have healing effects. Medicines have then been developed from concentrations of these active substances. However, each oil may contain up to 200 different chemical constituents. The interaction of these confers the 'power' to the oil, possibly also reducing potential adverse effects, which come as part of the package with synthetic medications. Having said this, oils used in aromatherapy also must be used appropriately to ensure optimal benefit and minimal adverse reactions.

Like so many doctors, I chose medicine as a career because I wanted to 'make people better'. Although educated in and practising in the science of allopathic medicine according to the Western orthodox model, I remained open to learning about any healing modality which would help my clients. In the early 1990s I became interested in the potential healing benefits of aromatherapy, having heard about positive experiences with clients suffering with a variety of conditions. In 1992–3 I studied aromatherapy under the expert guidance of the author of this book.

The interest in aromatherapy over the last decade, among both the general public and the medical fraternity, has spawned a plethora of books on the subject. However, not everyone who has an interest in the modality is able to study the subject in depth. What was needed was an easily readable book that would provide background information, including the origins of the therapy and the extraction of oils, the therapeutic properties and details of usage of the specific oils – with cautions where appropriate – together with reference to interesting collateral therapies which may well whet the appetite of those drawn to the natural approach to read further. The book should not only provide information about the wide range of ailments that might benefit from the aromatherapeutic approach but should endorse the benefits of allopathic medicine where appropriate, promoting aromatherapy as a 'complementary' rather than an 'alternative' therapeutic approach.

This latest edition has an expanded directory of oils and will be a valuable resource for all those interested in the subject of aromatherapy.

Dr Joan Kinder MA, MB, B.Chir (Cantab), MRCP, FRCPCH

Acknowledgments

I would like to express my gratitude to Dr Joan Kinder for her excellent foreword.

Contents

Meet the author

Welcome to *Change Your Mood with Aromatherapy*!

I have been practising and teaching complementary medicine since the 1980s. Initially trained in massage and aromatherapy, I was led by my enthusiasm and passion to study many other complementary therapies including osteopathy, reflexology, diet and nutrition, Indian head massage, sports massage, iridology, Bach Flower Remedies, crystal therapy, craniosacral therapy, meditation and healing ... and I am still learning!

During my career I have carried out tens of thousands of treatments and I continue to treat clients with a wide variety of conditions – physical, mental, emotional and spiritual. The results can still amaze both me and my clients.

In 1987 I established Beaumont College of Natural Medicine. Students from all over the world and from all walks of life come to study with me in small groups and it is a joy to inspire and nurture them and see their skills develop over the years.

I was commissioned to write my first two books in 1992 by Hodder & Stoughton – the Headway Lifeguides *Massage* and *Aromatherapy*. Since then I have written more than 20 books on aspects of complementary medicine which have been translated into many languages.

Over 20 years ago I established my own essential oil company with the aim of providing products of the highest quality and purity.

I now live in Somerset, UK, where I have set up the Beaumont Natural Health Centre in Wells near Bath. At my centre I teach professional training courses and offer a combination of therapies tailored to suit each individual's requirements.

Only got a minute?

Aromatherapy is a holistic therapy that uses essential oils to enhance health and vitality on all levels physical, mental, emotional and spiritual.

Essential oils may be used in numerous ways to create a healing aromatic environment and to prevent and treat common ailments.

Methods include:

► baths – 6 drops

► compresses – 6 drops

► gargles – 2 drops

► oil burners – 6 drops

► massage – 3 drops of essential oil to 10 ml carrier oil.

Essential oils are highly concentrated; they should be blended with a carrier oil rather than being used undiluted.

Just a few of the essential oils covered in this book can meet your everyday needs. Why not begin with:

- ► bergamot – treats anxiety and stress
- ► cajeput – ideal for coughs and colds
- ► chamomile – ideal for babies' and children's problems
- ► cypress – reduces fluid retention
- ► geranium – balances hormones, emotions and skin
- ► lavender – most versatile of all essential oils
- ► lemon – great pick-me-up, detoxifying and tonic
- ► peppermint – cooling, pain relieving and treats digestive problems
- ► rosemary – stimulates and restores, awakens the mind.

5 Only got five minutes?

Aromatherapy is a holistic therapy that uses essential oils to enhance health and vitality on all levels – physical, mental, emotional and spiritual.

Essential oils are obtained from many different parts of plants, e.g.:

- chamomile/rose – flowers
- peppermint/eucalyptus – leaves
- lemon/bergamot – fruits
- juniper – berries
- fennel – seeds
- ginger – root
- frankincense – gum.

The most widely used method of extracting essential oils is distillation. Expression and solvent extraction are also important methods.

Essential oils may be used in numerous ways to create a beautiful healing aromatic environment and to prevent and treat common ailments. Methods include:

Baths

Use 6 drops.

Simply fill the bath and add 6 drops of your chosen pure undiluted essential oil(s) into the water, agitating it thoroughly.

- Stress-buster – 2 drops each of geranium, lavender and ylang ylang.

Showers/footbaths/hand baths

Use 6 drops.

▶ To wake you up – sprinkle 2 drops each of black pepper/ lemon/rosemary onto a damp sponge or add the drops to an unperfumed shower gel (6 drops to 20 ml).
▶ For feel-good feet – 3 drops lavender and 3 drops peppermint in a bowl of hand-hot water. Soak your feet for about 10 minutes.
▶ To soothe painful and arthritic hands – 3 drops chamomile and 3 drops lavender in a bowl of hand-hot water. Soak your hands for about 10 minutes.

Compresses

Use 6 drops.

▶ To relieve a fever fill a small bowl with cold water and add 3 drops lavender and 3 drops peppermint. Soak up with a flannel (or other absorbent material). Apply the compress either to the forehead or the back of the neck.

Gargles/mouthwashes

Use 2 drops.

▶ To sweeten breath add 1 drop peppermint and 1 drop lemon to half a glass of water. Stir well, gargle and spit it out.

Steam inhalations

Use 3 drops.

▶ To clear the sinuses add 3 drops cajeput (or eucalyptus) to a bowl of hand-hot water, cover your head with a towel, lean over the bowl inhaling deeply for a few minutes, keeping your eyes closed to avoid irritation.

Oil burner

Use 6 drops.

▶ Fill the bowl on the top with water and sprinkle approximately 6 drops of essential oil into it. Light a nightlight candle and the oils will diffuse into the atmosphere (to repel insects use citronella).

Massage

Add 3 drops to 10 ml (approximately two teaspoons) carrier oil such as sweet almond oil.

▶ For constipation massage the abdomen gently in a clockwise direction using 3 drops marjoram and 3 drops rosemary.

Essential oils are highly concentrated and should not be used undiluted on the skin (except for lavender and tea tree for first aid purposes). Blend them with a cold-pressed, unrefined, additive-free carrier oil.

Sweet almond, apricot kernel and peach kernel all make good massage mediums – they are therapeutic, have a good texture (not too thick and sticky), absorb well and do not have a strong aroma that will mask the aroma of the essential oils.

More than 50 essential oils are covered in this book. Check out the main properties of 15 of them.

Bergamot

- ▶ Fresh, citrus, fruity aroma.
- ▶ Uplifting – antidepressant.
- ▶ Ideal for all states of anxiety, depression and stress-related disorders.
- ▶ Useful for digestive disorders especially when stress-related, e.g. anorexia.
- ▶ Use in a sitz bath to combat cystitis.

Cajeput

- ▶ Penetrating, medicinal aroma.
- ▶ Decongestive – stimulating – warming.
- ▶ Invaluable for the respiratory system as a chest rub and in inhalations.
- ▶ Clears the mind.
- ▶ Recommended for pain relief for aches, painful joints and sports injury.

Chamomile (Roman)

- ▶ Sweet, fresh, warm aroma.
- ▶ Balancing – calming – anti-inflammatory.
- ▶ A must-have oil for babies and children – colic, temper tantrums, etc.

- Ideal for skin that is inflamed, sensitive or prone to allergies.
- Recommended for PMT and the menopause.

Cypress

- Woody, reminiscent of pine needles.
- Astringent – fluid-reducing.
- Highly recommended for fluid retention and reducing varicose veins.
- Excellent for oily skin and excessive perspiration.
- Helps us to deal with change – e.g. menopause, bereavement.

Eucalyptus

- Camphor-like, penetrating aroma.
- Antiseptic – expectorant – pain-relieving – stimulating.
- Recommended for all respiratory problems.
- Due to its pain-relieving properties indicated for all aches and pains, arthritis and rheumatism.
- Combats mental exhaustion.

Frankincense

- Woody, spicy, balsamic aroma.
- Decongestive – healing – rejuvenating.
- Encourages the breathing to slow down and deepen.
- Frankincense allows past traumas to fade away and instils peace and calm.
- Rejuvenates mature skin and helps to prevent ageing.

Geranium

- Sweet, rosy aroma.
- Antidepressant – balancing – uplifting.
- Geranium gently balances the hormones and is excellent for the menopause and PMT.
- Dispels anxiety and depression and will help to balance all types of skin.

Ginger

- Aromatic, hot, spicy aroma.
- Digestive – fiery – stimulant.
- A warming oil effective for poor circulation.
- Ginger is excellent for all digestive problems especially nausea and is also indicated for all aches and pains. It sharpens the senses and aids concentration.

Jasmine

- Exotic, floral, heady, sensual aroma.
- Antidepressant – aphrodisiac – euphoric.
- A wonderful oil for all problems of the nervous system, releasing anxiety, lifting sadness and inducing optimism and confidence.
- Highly recommended for childbirth and also a renowned aphrodisiac.

Lavender

- Sweet, floral, herbaceous aroma.
- Balancing – calming – healing.

- ▶ Most versatile of all essential oils and a must-have for the first aid kit.
- ▶ Lavender harmonizes the nervous system and relieves stress and anxiety.
- ▶ Boosts the circulation and immune system and relieves aches and pains.
- ▶ Lavender is useful for all skin problems.

Lemon

- ▶ Clean, crisp, fruity, refreshing aroma.
- ▶ Alkaline – detoxifying – tonic.
- ▶ Stimulates and cleanses the circulatory system and useful for varicose veins.
- ▶ Lemon is highly recommended for the digestion – it relieves acidity and is ideal for detoxification.
- ▶ It may be applied neat to warts and verrucae.
- ▶ Lemon clears the mind.

Peppermint

- ▶ Cool, piercing, menthol aroma.
- ▶ Cooling – digestive – pain-relieving – stimulating.
- ▶ Recommended for all digestive problems.
- ▶ Peppermint is excellent for general pain relief and exerts a cooling and anaesthetic action when used on headaches, migraine and fevers.

Rose

- ▶ Sweet, heady, intoxicating, heavenly aroma.
- ▶ Aphrodisiac – rejuvenating – uplifting.

- This 'queen' of oils has a remarkable effect on all female problems. The exquisite, luxurious aroma has a profound effect on the emotions, dissolving psychological pain and helping a woman feel feminine and positive.

Rosemary

- Clean, camphoraceous, herbaceous aroma.
- Invigorating – restorative – stimulating.
- An excellent tonic for the circulation. Highly recommended for the digestion and for muscles and joints.
- Rosemary activates and enlivens the brain promoting clarity.

Ylang ylang

- Exotic, heady, sweet, seductive aroma.
- Antidepressant – aphrodisiac – euphoric.
- A sensuous oil that provides a very powerful aphrodisiac.
- Ylang ylang is deeply relaxing and relieves anxiety, anger and fear and creates a sense of euphoria.
- Excellent for skin care.

10 Only got ten minutes?

Aromatherapy is a holistic therapy that uses essential oils to enhance health and vitality on all levels – physical, mental, emotional and spiritual.

Essential oils are obtained from many different parts of plants, e.g.:

- ▶ chamomile/rose – flowers
- ▶ peppermint/eucalyptus – leaves
- ▶ lemon/bergamot – fruits
- ▶ juniper – berries
- ▶ fennel – seeds
- ▶ ginger – root
- ▶ frankincense – gum.

The most widely used method of extracting essential oils is distillation. Expression and solvent extraction are also important methods.

Expression is reserved exclusively for members of the citrus family such as bergamot, grapefruit, lemon, lime and mandarin.

Solvent extraction does not yield essential oils – this process produces 'absolutes' and 'resinoids'. This technique is used for higher yield or to extract oils that cannot be obtained by any other process.

Essential oils may be used in numerous ways to create a beautiful healing aromatic environment and to prevent and treat common ailments. Methods include:

Baths

Use 6 drops.

Simply fill the bath and add 6 drops of your chosen pure undiluted essential oil(s) into the water, agitating it thoroughly.

▶ Stress-buster – 2 drops each of geranium, lavender and ylang ylang.

Showers/footbaths/hand baths

Use 6 drops.

▶ To wake you up sprinkle 2 drops each of black pepper/lemon/rosemary onto a damp sponge or add the drops to an unperfumed shower gel. (6 drops to 20 ml).
▶ For feel-good feet – 3 drops lavender and 3 drops peppermint in a bowl of hand-hot water. Soak your feet for about 10 minutes.
▶ To soothe painful and arthritic hands – 3 drops chamomile and 3 drops lavender in a bowl of hand-hot water. Soak your hands for about 10 minutes.

Compresses

Use 6 drops.

▶ To relieve a fever fill a small bowl with cold water and add 3 drops lavender and 3 drops peppermint. Soak up with a flannel (or other absorbent material). Apply the compress either to the forehead or to the back of the neck.

Gargles/mouthwashes

Use 2 drops.

▶ To sweeten breath add 1 drop peppermint and 1 drop lemon to half a glass of water. Stir well, gargle and spit it out.

Steam inhalations

Use 3 drops.

▶ To clear the sinuses add 3 drops cajeput (or eucalyptus) to a bowl of hand-hot water, cover your head with a towel, lean over the bowl inhaling deeply for a few minutes, keeping your eyes closed to avoid irritation.

Oil burner

Use 6 drops.

▶ Fill the bowl on the top with water and sprinkle approximately 6 drops of essential oil into it. Light a nightlight candle and the oils will diffuse into the atmosphere. (To repel insects use citronella.)

Massage

Add 3 drops to 10 ml (approximately two teaspoons) carrier oil such as sweet almond oil.

▶ For constipation, massage the abdomen gently in a clockwise direction using 3 drops marjoram and 3 drops rosemary.

Essential oils are highly concentrated and should not be used undiluted on the skin (except for lavender and tea tree and for first aid purposes). Blend them with a cold-pressed, unrefined, additive-free carrier oil.

Sweet almond, apricot kernel and peach kernel all make good massage mediums – they are therapeutic, have a good texture (not too thick and sticky), absorb well and do not have a strong aroma that will mask the aroma of the essential oils.

These carrier oils may be used on their own or you can blend them with thicker, more viscous oils to increase their therapeutic value. For instance, avocado pear, calendula, jojoba and wheatgerm. A blend could be 80 ml sweet almond, and 5 ml each of avocado, jojoba, calendula and wheatgerm.

More than 50 essential oils are covered in this book. Check out the main properties of 25 of them.

Bergamot

- ▶ Fresh, citrus, fruity aroma.
- ▶ Uplifting – antidepressant.
- ▶ Ideal for all states of anxiety, depression and stress-related disorders.
- ▶ Useful for digestive disorders especially when stress-related, e.g. anorexia.
- ▶ Use in a sitz bath to combat cystitis.

Cajeput

- ▶ Penetrating, medicinal aroma.
- ▶ Decongestive – stimulating – warming.
- ▶ Invaluable for the respiratory system as a chest rub and in inhalations.

- Clears the mind.
- Recommended for pain relief for aches, painful joints and sports injury.

Chamomile (Roman)

- Sweet, fresh, warm aroma.
- Balancing – calming – anti-inflammatory.
- A must-have oil for babies and children – colic, temper tantrums, etc.
- Ideal for skin that is inflamed, sensitive or prone to allergies.
- Recommended for PMT and the menopause.

Clary sage

- Sweet, heady, floral aroma.
- Euphoric – intoxicating – relaxing.
- Indicated for all stress-related disorders as it has a euphoric-sedative effect.
- Clary sage induces a sense of well-being and creates a padding between you and the outside world.

Cypress

- Woody, reminiscent of pine needles.
- Astringent – fluid-reducing.
- Highly recommended for fluid retention and reducing varicose veins.
- Excellent for oily skin and excessive perspiration.
- Helps us to deal with change – e.g. menopause, bereavement.

Eucalyptus

▶ Camphor-like penetrating aroma.
▶ Antiseptic – expectorant – pain-relieving – stimulating.
▶ Recommended for all respiratory problems.
▶ Due to its pain relieving properties indicated for all aches and pains, arthritis and rheumatism.
▶ Combats mental exhaustion.

Fennel

▶ Aniseed-like, strong, sweet aroma.
▶ Detoxifying – digestive – energizing.
▶ Excellent for cleansing the digestive system as well as the other systems too. Fennel is a helpful aid for slimming. Fennel is energizing and induces courage and strength in the face of seemingly impossible hurdles.

Frankincense

▶ Woody, spicy, balsamic aroma.
▶ Decongestive – healing – rejuvenating.
▶ Encourages the breathing to slow down and deepen.
▶ Frankincense allows past traumas to fade away and instils peace and calm.
▶ Rejuvenates mature skin and helps to prevent ageing.

Geranium

▶ Sweet, rosy aroma.
▶ Antidepressant – balancing – uplifting.

- ▶ Geranium gently balances the hormones and is excellent for the menopause and PMT.
- ▶ It dispels anxiety and depression and will help to balance all types of skin.

Ginger

- ▶ Aromatic, hot, spicy aroma.
- ▶ Digestive – fiery – stimulant.
- ▶ A warming oil effective for poor circulation.
- ▶ Ginger is excellent for all digestive problems especially nausea and is also indicated for all aches and pains. It sharpens the senses and aids concentration.

Jasmine

- ▶ Exotic, floral, heady, sensual aroma.
- ▶ Antidepressant – aphrodisiac – euphoric.
- ▶ A wonderful oil for all problems of the nervous system, releasing anxiety, lifting sadness and inducing optimism and confidence.
- ▶ Highly recommended for childbirth and also a renowned aphrodisiac.

Juniper berry

- ▶ Fresh, woody, pine-needle aroma.
- ▶ Cleansing – fluid-reducing – purifying.
- ▶ A classic remedy for purification of body, mind and spirit.
- ▶ Juniper encourages elimination on all levels.
- ▶ Juniper is excellent for fluid retention and as an overall tonic.

Lavender

▶ Sweet, floral, herbaceous aroma.
▶ Balancing – calming – healing.
▶ Most versatile of all essential oils and a must-have for the first aid kit.
▶ Lavender harmonizes the nervous system and relieves stress and anxiety.
▶ Boosts the circulation, immune system and relieves aches and pains.
▶ Lavender is useful for all skin problems.

Lemon

▶ Clean, crisp, fruity, refreshing aroma.
▶ Alkaline – detoxifying – tonic.
▶ Stimulates and cleanses the circulatory system and useful for varicose veins.
▶ Lemon is highly recommended for the digestion – it relieves acidity and is ideal for detoxification.
▶ It may be applied neat to warts and verrucae.
▶ Lemon clears the mind.

Mandarin

▶ Sweet, floral, tangy aroma.
▶ Balancing – joyful – revitalizing.
▶ A therapeutic oil for young children, in pregnancy, and for people who are frail or elderly.
▶ Mandarin is a gentle oil which relieves stress and anxiety and engenders joy and hopefulness.

Marjoram (sweet)

- ▶ Sweet, warming, camphoraceous aroma.
- ▶ Calming – digestive – sedative – warming.
- ▶ An excellent oil for improving the circulation and relieving chilblains.
- ▶ Marjoram alleviates pain and stiffness in the joints and is recommended for constipation and digestive disorders.
- ▶ It has a warming and comforting effect on the emotions, easing grief and sadness.

Myrrh

- ▶ Warm, balsamic, medicinal aroma.
- ▶ Anticatarrhal – healing – rejuvenating.
- ▶ A highly effective oil for respiratory problems such as catarrh and coughs and renowned as a gargle for sore throats, mouth ulcers and gum disorders.
- ▶ Myrrh heals cracked and chapped skin and rejuvenates mature and wrinkled skin.

Neroli

- ▶ Fresh, floral, haunting, light aroma.
- ▶ Antidepressant – aphrodisiac – stress-relieving.
- ▶ Invaluable for all nervous problems, chronic and short-term anxiety and panic attacks.
- ▶ Neroli lifts depression and instils confidence and positivity.
- ▶ Its aphrodisiacal properties make it ideal for all sexual problems.

Patchouli

- Sweet, earthy, musty aroma.
- Antidepressant – rejuvenating – soothing.
- Popular in the 1960s due to its ability to instil peace, calm and love, patchouli is beneficial for all stress-related problems.
- Patchouli encourages the regeneration of skin cells and is recommended for mature skin.

Peppermint

- Cool, piercing, menthol aroma.
- Cooling – digestive – pain-relieving – stimulating.
- Recommended for all digestive problems.
- Peppermint is excellent for general pain relief and exerts a cooling and anaesthetic action when used on headaches, migraine and fevers.

Rose

- Sweet, heady, intoxicating, heavenly aroma.
- Aphrodisiac – rejuvenating – uplifting.
- This 'queen' of oils has a remarkable effect on all female problems. The exquisite, luxurious aroma has a profound effect on the emotions, dissolving psychological pain and helps a woman feel feminine and positive.

Rosemary

- Clean, camphoraceous, herbaceous aroma.
- Invigorating – restorative – stimulating.

- An excellent tonic for the circulation. Highly recommended for the digestion and for muscles and joints.
- Rosemary activates and enlivens the brain promoting clarity.

Sandalwood

- Sweet, warm, woody, lingering aroma.
- Healing – soothing – uplifting.
- Renowned for its balancing effect on the nervous system, gently soothing away anxiety and tension.
- Sandalwood is used extensively for skin complaints, especially dry and dehydrated skin.

Tea tree

- Sharp, strong, medicinal aroma.
- Antifungal – antiseptic – first aid.
- Recommended as an immune-booster to combat repeated infections.
- A must-have for the first aid kit, tea tree can be applied neat to warts and verrucae and is indicated for athlete's foot, cuts, itching, spots and sweaty or smelly feet.
- Useful for mouth ulcers and cold sores too.

Ylang ylang

- Exotic, heady, sweet, seductive aroma.
- Antidepressant – aphrodisiac – euphoric.
- A sensuous oil that provides a very powerful aphrodisiac.
- Ylang ylang is deeply relaxing and relieves anxiety, anger and fear and creates a sense of euphoria.
- Excellent for skin care.

Introduction

Aromatherapy has become one of the fastest growing natural healing arts in the UK. It is rapidly gaining respect from orthodox medical practitioners, and qualified clinical aromatherapists now work not only from their own private practices but also in hospitals, hospices and surgeries.

The art of aromatherapy uses pure essential oils which are extracted from various parts of plants and trees. These natural, aromatic, liquid substances, often considered to be the 'life force' or 'soul' of plants, are endowed with a whole host of therapeutic properties. They are remarkably versatile and may be used in various ways. This book aims to show you how to use essential oils safely and effectively on your friends and family without creating harmful side-effects, unlike many chemical drugs. The information contained within these pages will also be very useful to the student or practising aromatherapist.

Aromatherapy is a holistic therapy which can be used to promote physical, mental and spiritual health equilibrium. It forms part of a holistic healing regime which involves searching for the root causes of an illness, rather than its symptoms, and awakening the body's innate ability to heal itself, leading to a state of balance. Aromatherapy involves far more than the application of essential oils. To achieve 'whole healing', factors such as diet and lifestyle must always be considered.

A great deal of this book is devoted to the 'holistic' treatment of various conditions. I have indicated not only which essential oils should be selected on a physical, emotional and spiritual level but also which Bach Flower Remedies may be appropriate to enable us to treat the person rather than the disease. These remedies, I believe, are a valuable accompaniment to essential oils. They aim to balance our negative states of mind, such as worry, depression and fear, which are so depleting to our immune systems and ultimately can lead to serious disease. I have also included dietary advice for each condition, which is vital if true healing is to take place. Where appropriate I have suggested other courses of action which can enhance and support the aromatherapy treatment.

Since I have stepped into the world of essential oils, my life has been completely transformed. I do hope that you will allow aromatherapy to become part of your daily life and that this book will encourage you to learn more about these fascinating, healing, essential oils which can help you to achieve balance of mind, body and spirit.

1

The history of aromatherapy

In this chapter you will learn:
- *about the origins and development of aromatherapy.*

Plants have been employed for medicinal purposes since the dawn of mankind. Primitive people relied very much on their instincts to keep them alive. By using their sense of smell and drawing on experience they were able to acquire knowledge of how certain plants had the capacity to heal and cure ailments and diseases. When they are sick, animals too instinctively search for plants which can heal and relieve their symptoms.

Early civilizations

In the caves of Lascaux in the Dordogne region of France there are cave paintings which depict the use of plants for healing and medicinal purposes. Archaeologists estimate that these paintings date back as far as 18000 BC.

A terracotta 'still' which experts believe to be 5,000 years old is housed in the Taxila Museum in Pakistan. This still would have been employed for making aromatic waters and even perhaps for the production of essential oils. It is believed to have belonged to the ancient Indus or Arab civilizations. This is a curious phenomenon since distillation was thought to have been 'invented' only 1,000 years ago. There is no other evidence of the use of distillation from 5000 to 1000 BC. It can therefore be assumed that 5,000 years ago ancient civilizations must have been far more advanced than was previously thought.

EGYPT

I believe that aromatherapy was born in ancient Egypt, and plant medicine dates back to at least 3000 BC. There is much evidence to suggest that aromatics formed a part of Egyptian daily life. Around 3000 BC the oldest known pyramid in Egypt, the 'Step Pyramid', was built by King Zoser at Saqqara. His chief architect was the genius Imhotep who was a renowned physician as well as an astronomer and scribe. Imhotep did a great deal to advance medical knowledge at this time and he is sometimes referred to as the 'grandfather of aromatherapy'.

The Papyrus of Ebers (1550 BC), one of the few surviving medical papyri, reveals the widespread and frequent use of aromatics in Egyptian medicine. From the papyrus it is apparent that aromatics were used both externally and internally to combat health problems. Egyptian priests prescribed medicinal wines for all sorts of conditions. Inhalations were taken for respiratory problems. Sitz baths and douches were recommended for gynaecological disorders. Gargles were employed for problems with the mouth and gums, and ointments were prepared for diseases of the skin.

The ordinary Egyptians used aromatics in their cooking for health purposes. Garlic, for instance, was highly prized for its ability to ward off disease and to prevent the outbreak of epidemics. Other herbs and spices used include aniseed, caraway, mint, marjoram and parsley.

The Egyptian perfumers were highly skilled and they formulated the famous 'Kyphi' – a favourite perfume and incense. It was a blend of 16 aromatics. The exact ingredients of Kyphi are unknown but it is thought to have contained calamus, cinnamon, frankincense, henna, juniper and myrrh, among others.

Kyphi was a popular item in the Egyptian home and was not only employed as a perfume and burned as an incense but also presented as a medicine. It was inhaled during meditations to heighten spiritual awareness. Its ingredients encouraged new levels of consciousness. Frankincense was also used to increase spiritual and psychic awareness. It is fascinating that when the tomb of Tutankhamen, who ruled from 1361 to 1352 BC, was opened in 1922, in one of the sealed flasks was an unguent which still had an aroma – despite the fact it was over 3300 years old. Frankincense was one of the aromatics it contained.

Insight

Not only were the Egyptians aware of the health benefits of essential oils for physical problems, they also knew of their effects on the emotions. Perfumes were formulated for the pharaohs to uplift the spirits, dispel nervousness, encourage love, bring tranquillity and induce aggression for the purposes of war.

Perfumes and religion were closely connected. The Egyptians adorned their gods with scented oils; gods and goddesses had fragrances dedicated to them and the statues were sometimes anointed. For instance, myrrh was dedicated to the moon and frankincense to the sun god, Ra. Aromatics were burned during religious ceremonies as offerings to the deities. (The Latin *per fumum* means 'through smoke'.)

Wealthy Egyptian women would indulge themselves in an aromatherapy massage after a bath. Their slave girls would apply the oils which rejuvenated and perfumed the skin. Cedarwood oil was a particular favourite. Egyptian women even knew about contraception. Aromatic mixtures were blended together and placed in the vagina to act as spermicides.

The Egyptians strongly believed in reincarnation and the afterlife, and when we think of Egyptians we always associate them with the process of mummification. They went to tremendous lengths in their embalming procedures and they really were experts.

They removed many of the major organs, including the brain which was hooked out through the nostrils, and the abdominal viscera were also taken out. Myrrh, cassia, galbanum and other aromatic substances were employed to fill up the cavities. The blood was drained out and then the body was bathed in natron (a sodium carbonate solution). The body was left for approximately 70 days and then wrapped in bandages which had been soaked with various aromatics including cedarwood oil. Each embalmer would have his own particular recipe. The formulations were remarkably effective at preserving human flesh and even now, after thousands of years, mummies have been discovered in a wonderful state of preservation. These elaborate procedures, of course, were employed only for the embalming of high priests and pharaohs.

The Nile Valley became known as the 'Cradle of Medicine'. Medicinal plants such as cedarwood, cinnamon, frankincense and myrrh were transported to this area to grow. When the Jews began their exodus from Egypt to Israel in about 1240 BC they took with them much knowledge and many precious gums and oils.

Insight
In the Old and New Testaments of the Bible there are numerous references to oils, including, calamus, cassia, cinnamon, hyssop and olive, and, of course, frankincense and myrrh were offered to Jesus Christ at his birth.

CHINA

Aromatic herbs and massage were used in China long before the birth of Christ. Along the Yellow River 5000 years ago the Chinese were using mugwort leaves and calamus roots for hygiene purposes. Emperor Shen Nung's medical text *Herbal* dates back to about 2700 BC and it contains details of 365 plants. Emperor Huang Ti is credited with *The Yellow Emperor's Classic of Internal Medicine* (2650 BC). In this work aromatic medicines and massage are referred to on several occasions. The book also forms much of the basis for acupuncture.

INDIA

In India, plants and plant extracts were being employed from at least 3000 BC. The oldest form of Indian medicine is known as Ayurvedic medicine. It uses many different massage techniques, pressure points and also essential oils. One of the oldest known Indian books, the *Vedas*, mentions basil, cinnamon, coriander, ginger, myrrh and sandalwood.

THE GREEKS

The ancient Greeks played a very important part in aromatic medicine, developing the knowledge acquired from the Egyptians.

The most renowned Greek physician was Hippocrates (460–370 BC), who became known as the 'Father of Medicine'. He wrote in his *Aphorisms* that 'aromatic baths are useful in the treatment of female disorders' and advocated their use on a daily basis for all.

Insight

Hippocrates, the 'Father of Medicine', adopted a holistic approach. He claimed: 'The way to health is to have an aromatic bath and scented massage every day'.

The Greek philosopher and physician Asclepiades (200 BC) believed in gentle therapies such as bathing, massage, music, perfume and wine. He was opposed to the use of purgatives and emetics which were so popular at that time. Theophrastus, the famous Greek botanist, advocated the use of perfumes, plasters and poultices for medicinal purposes. He had noticed that oils which are applied externally can affect the internal organs. Another Greek was Megallus, who formulated a successful preparation containing cassia, cinnamon and myrrh known as 'Megaleion', renowned throughout Greece.

THE ROMANS

Pedanius Dioscorides of Anazarbus wrote a five-volume book known as *De Materia Medica* in the first century AD. One of the volumes is full of information regarding the uses of plants and aromatics. Cypress, juniper, marjoram and myrrh are mentioned among the 500 plants described in this study. He mentions Kyphi, claiming that it is calming and helps to relieve asthma attacks. Other formulae include 'Amarakinon' to treat haemorrhoids and menstrual difficulties, 'Susinon' to treat fluid retention and 'Nardinon muron' for coughs and colds. A great deal of our present knowledge of medicinal herbs comes from Dioscorides.

The Romans adored perfumes and aromatic oils and used them for massage and scenting their hair and clothing. In Rome the *hetairi*, or prostitutes, used scent lavishly. Galen, the physician to the gladiators, prepared ointments and he also produced a 'cold cream'.

As the Roman soldiers marched into battle they carried myrrh with them to heal their wounds. Their knowledge of the healing properties of plants spread throughout their growing Empire. Wherever they went they collected and planted seeds. In Britain, for instance, herbs such as parsley, sage, fennel, rosemary and thyme were planted.

AVICENNA

Born in Persia, the physician and scholar Avicenna (AD 980–1037) is credited with the invention of distillation. There was already a crude type of distillation in operation, but Avicenna refined it by extending the length of the cooling pipe and forming it into a coil. This enabled the condensation of steam and vaporized essence to be far more efficient. Rose water made from *Rosa centifolia* became popular. The Persians exported it to China, Europe and India where it was used for medicinal and culinary purposes. Perfumes were formulated using roses, lilies, narcissi and violets.

Avicenna wrote almost 100 books throughout his life. His most renowned work is the *Canon of Medicine*. This book was used as a standard reference text by many medical schools for 500 years up until the middle of the sixteenth century. Avicenna mentions many essential oils including chamomile, cinnamon, dill and peppermint.

The medieval Crusaders who fought in the Holy Land brought back knowledge of herbal medicines and perfumes handed down from the Romans.

The Middle Ages

Religious orders cultivated their own aromatic plants – in the twelfth century the German Abbess Hildegarde was well known for growing lavender.

In the Middle Ages lavender and other herbs made up into bouquets were used as protection against plagues. Frankincense and pine were burnt in the streets in the fourteenth century. Basil, chamomile, lavender, melissa and thyme were strewn on the ground and chamomile lawns became popular. Perfumes were used widely in England as people hardly ever washed themselves, and the perfumes masked unpleasant natural body odours.

During the sixteenth century many books were written on distillation, many of them in German. Alchemy – the practice of trying to transform base metal into gold – was widespread. In 1576, the Swiss physician and alchemist Paracelsus wrote the *Great Surgery Book*. He claimed that the role of alchemy was not to turn base metals into gold but instead to develop medicines, especially medicines from plants.

In 1597 the German Hieronymous Braunschweig published his book called *New Vollkommen Distillierbuch* containing references to 25 essential oils.

Throughout the Renaissance period essential oils were widely used and botany was part of the study of medicine.

The seventeenth, eighteenth and nineteenth centuries

Many English herbalists emerged during the seventeenth century. The most renowned herbalists include John Parkinson, John Gerarde and Nicholas Culpeper. In 1653 Culpeper wrote his famous *Complete Herbal*. The plague wreaked havoc once more and aromatic herbs were popular. The perfumers enjoyed an immunity to the plague because they were surrounded by essential oils. Essential oils were being used in mainstream medicine for a host of internal and external diseases.

Insight

During the eighteenth century the use of essential oils was widespread. Practically all herbalists and some doctors were using essential oils. Potions were mixed up by apothecaries – each had his own still.

Scientists of the nineteenth century identified some of the chemical constituents of oils and gave them names such as 'geraniol' and 'citronellol'. Unfortunately this led to the development of synthetic copies of the main constituents of the oils. The use of herbs and essential oils declined greatly as the drug companies started to flourish. Synthetic drugs, sadly, can produce numerous side-effects and can be toxic and harmful.

The twentieth century

The birth of modern aromatherapy can be attributed to the French chemist René Maurice Gattefossé. It was Gattefossé who coined the word 'aromatherapy' in 1937 with the publication of his book *Aromathérapie*. It is said that after burning his hand in an experiment, he plunged it into the nearest liquid which happened to contain lavender oil. He used essential oils on the wounds of soldiers who were injured during the First World War.

Other chemists were also investigating the use of essential oils. In Australia, Penfold and others were researching the benefits of tea tree oil. In Italy, doctors Giovanni Gatti and Renato Cayola discovered the psychotherapeutic effects of essential oils – such as jasmine and lemon.

French doctor Jean Valnet, an army surgeon who had been influenced by the work of Gattefossé, made an enormous impact on the aromatherapy world.

Insight

Jean Valnet's book *Aromathérapie*, published in 1964, is regarded by many as the 'aromatherapist's bible'. It is essential reading for all those studying a professional aromatherapy course.

Valnet had used essential oils for treating war wounds and after the war he continued to use essential oils. He taught other members of the medical profession about the therapeutic effects of essential oils. In France some doctors study aromatherapy and prescribe essential oils.

Madame Marguerite Maury (1895–1964) introduced aromatherapy into Britain in the late 1950s. She applied the essential oils, diluted in a carrier oil, using massage techniques. She taught her techniques to beauty therapists and wrote a book called *The Secret of Life and Youth* which is concerned with rejuvenation.

Nowadays aromatherapy is becoming an increasingly popular therapy for a wide range of ailments. Many of us now regularly use essential oils for our health and healing. Aromatherapy is practised by professionally qualified clinical aromatherapists in hospitals, clinics, hospices and surgeries. The demand for aromatherapy is growing rapidly.

TEST YOUR KNOWLEDGE

1 The 'Father of Medicine' is considered to be:
  a Hippocrates
  b Imhotep
  c Avicenna
  d Emperor Huang Ti

2 What was Kyphi?

3 Which country does Ayurvedic medicine originate from?

4 Distillation was invented by:
  a Hippocrates
  b Avicenna
  c Dioscorides
  d Galen

5 Why were herbs used during the plagues?

6 In 1937 the word 'aromatherapy' was coined by:
  a Jean Valnet
  b René Maurice Gattefossé

2

Extracting the oils

In this chapter you will learn:
* *the main methods of extracting essential oils.*

There are several methods of obtaining aromatic substances from plant material, most of which I have described below. But strictly speaking, essential oils are only those obtained by distillation or expression.

Insight

Essential oils are extracted from many different parts of plants. For example rose and chamomile are extracted from the flowers, peppermint and eucalyptus from the leaves, lemon and bergamot from the fruits, juniper from the berries, fennel from the seeds, ginger from the root and frankincense from the gum. In the A–Z of essential oils the methods of extraction and the part used is given.

Distillation

Distillation is the most widely used and the most economical method of extracting essential oils. Many historians attribute the discovery of distillation to Avicenna, the Persian physician and scholar (see Chapter 1), although possibly the Egyptians were aware of the primitive process. There is a great deal of skill involved in the process of distillation if the precious essential oil is not to be lost or changed in its composition. Some plants are distilled immediately after harvesting, whereas others may be left for a few days or even dried prior to extraction.

In distillation, the plant material is heated, either by placing it in water which is brought to the boil or by passing steam through it. The heat and steam cause the cell structure of the plant material to burst and break down, thus freeing the essential oils. The essential oil molecules and steam are carried along a pipe and channelled through a cooling tank, where they return to liquid form and are collected in a vat. The emerging liquid is a mixture of oil and water, and since essential oils are not water soluble they can be easily separated from the water and siphoned off. Essential oils which are lighter than water will float on the surface, whereas heavier oils, such as clove, will sink.

Insight

The water travelling around the distillation plant becomes impregnated with aroma and is recycled, and may be used as perfumed water such as lavender water or rose water. Rose water in particular is an excellent toner for the face.

During the process of distillation only the extremely small volatile molecules are able to evaporate. Essential oils which contain a high proportion of the smallest (most volatile) of these molecules are referred to as 'top notes'. Those which are composed mostly of the heaviest (least volatile) molecules are known as 'base notes'. Essential oils which are in between are called 'middle notes'.

Top note oils are the most volatile – the aroma disappears within 24 hours. Examples are basil, grapefruit, lemon, lime and eucalyptus. They tend to be stimulating and uplifting.

Middle note oils have an aroma which lasts for two to three days. Examples are chamomile, geranium and lavender. They are generally balancing and primarily affect the general metabolism and the systems of the body such as digestion and menstruation.

Base note oils are the least volatile – the aroma will last at least one week. Examples are frankincense, myrrh, neroli, patchouli and vetivert. They have a relaxing and sedative quality.

The first distillation is usually the best quality. If essential oils are redistilled this process is known as 'rectification'. The second and subsequent distillations will produce a cheaper oil unsuitable for aromatherapy.

Expression

This method is reserved exclusively for members of the citrus family such as bergamot, grapefruit, lemon, lime, mandarin and orange. The essence yielded is found in small sacs which are located under the surface of the rind. This process was originally carried out using simple hand pressure. The citrus essence was squeezed from the rinds and then collected in a sponge which, once saturated, was squeezed into a bucket. Why not try hand pressing the rind of a citrus fruit yourself? You can have your own hand expression plant in your kitchen!

Due to the labour costs involved, the majority of citrus oil is now expressed using mechanical presses. A great deal of essential oil of orange is produced in the United States in fruit-juice factories. However, this is not the best oil to use as the crops are treated with pesticides and chemical fertilizers which contaminate the essence. Citrus oils for therapeutic aromatherapy use are best obtained from organically or naturally grown fruit. The benefit of the expression process is that the essential oils are not subjected to heat.

Unfortunately some citrus oil factories distil the peel after expression in order to release more oil. Obviously this essential oil is of an inferior quality but it is often added to the expressed essential oil to increase the quantity and thus make more profit.

Insight

Citrus oils are great pick-me-ups and can be used in the morning to wake you up or at the end of a long hard day to revitalize and uplift. Sprinkle six drops into your bath, agitating thoroughly. Stay in the bath for about 15 minutes and notice how rejuvenated you feel.

Solvent extraction

The process of solvent extraction does not yield essential oils. This method is employed for flowers, gums and resins and it produces 'absolutes' and 'resinoids'. The technique is used for higher yield or to extract oils that cannot be obtained by any other process. Jasmine, for example, is adversely affected by hot water and steam.

ABSOLUTES

To yield an absolute, the aromatic plant material (flowers, leaves, etc.) is extracted by hydrocarbon solvents such as benzene or hexane. The plant material is covered with the solvent and slowly heated to dissolve the aromatic molecules. The solvent extracts the odour and then the solvent is filtered off to produce a 'concrete'. A concrete is a solid, wax-like substance containing about 50 per cent wax and 50 per cent volatile oil such as jasmine.

To obtain the absolute the concrete is mixed with pure alcohol to dissolve out the aromatic molecules, and then chilled. This mixture is filtered to eliminate waste products and to separate out insoluble waxes. The alcohol is evaporated off gently under vacuum. The thick, viscous, coloured liquid known as the absolute is left behind.

This method is widely used for rose, jasmine and neroli. A trace of the solvent, however, will always remain. Therefore an absolute can never be as pure as an essential oil which has been extracted via the process of distillation. Absolutes are sometimes adulterated because of their high price. Take care to always buy from a reputable supplier.

Insight

Rose otto is extracted by steam distillation of the fresh petals whereas Rose absolute is extracted by solvent extraction. Rose otto is purer and this is reflected in its higher price.

RESINOIDS

Solvent extraction can also be used for gums and resins to produce resinoids. Resins are the solid/semi-solid substances which exude naturally from a tree or plant that has been damaged. Commercially, resins are obtained by cutting into the bark or stem, and the gum-like substance hardens once it is exposed to the air.

The natural resinous material is extracted with a hydrocarbon solvent such as petroleum ether, hexane or alcohol. These solvents are then filtered off and subsequently removed by distillation.

A resinoid remains where a hydrocarbon solvent has been used (e.g. benzoin resinoid). If an alcohol solvent has been used then an absolute resin is produced (e.g. frankincense and myrrh resin absolutes may be extracted from the crude oleo resin gum – both, however, may be extracted by steam distillation to produce an essential oil).

Resinoids are often employed by perfume manufacturers as fixatives to prolong the aroma of a fragrance (as are concretes).

Enfleurage

The process of enfleurage also yields an absolute, although this method is virtually obsolete nowadays. It is very time consuming and labour intensive and, therefore, highly expensive.

Formerly this was the main method of extraction for delicate flowers such as jasmine which continue to produce perfume even after they have been picked. It involves the use of purified odourless cold fat which is spread over sheets of glass, mounted in large rectangular wooden frames. Flowers are strewn upon this layer of fat which absorbs the essential oil. After approximately a day, the flowers are removed to be replaced by fresh flowers. This process is repeated many times – even beyond two months – until the fat is saturated. This fragrance-saturated fat is known as a 'pomade'. The pomade is washed in alcohol and then treated. The alcohol evaporates first and the pure absolute is produced.

Carbon dioxide extraction

This relatively new method was introduced only in the 1980s. The price is high because the equipment used is expensive. The process has been designed for the perfume industry. Oils which are extracted utilizing carbon dioxide are supposed to be superior, pure and very close to the natural essential oil as it exists in the plant – and they are completely free of residues of carbon dioxide.

The prices are too high at the moment to be of value to the aromatherapist. However, as the costs are reduced and production increases they may become available. Research would be necessary to evaluate their therapeutic benefits since the composition of the essential oil is different.

Hydrodiffusion/percolation

Hydrodiffusion or percolation is the most modern method of extraction. This process is faster than distillation, and the equipment is much more simple than that used for carbon dioxide extraction. Steam spray is passed through the plant material (which is suspended on a grid) from above. The emerging liquid composed of oil and condensed steam is then cooled. The result is a mixture of essential oil and water (as in the distillation process) which can be easily separated. Although this method is promising, research is necessary to evaluate the place of these oils in aromatherapy.

Maceration

For this process plants are placed into a vat of warm vegetable oil which causes the plant cells to rupture, enabling the absorption of the essential oils. The vat is then agitated for several days. The resulting oil is filtered and bottled, and is ready for use as a massage medium. Examples of macerated oils are calendula, carrot and hypericum.

Insight

Why not try to make your own macerated oils at home? Half fill a glass jar with your chosen plant material (e.g. lemon balm). Add warm, good quality vegetable oil to fill up the jar. Screw the top on the jar and store it in a warm place for a week or so; remember to shake the jar daily. Finally, filter off the plant material, rebottle and label.

TEST YOUR KNOWLEDGE

1 *What is the most widely used method of extraction?*

2 *Which method is used for citrus oils?*

3 *Which method of extraction produces an absolute?*

4 *Why are resinoids employed by perfume manufacturers?*

5 *Why is enfleurage no longer used as a method of extraction?*

3

Buying, storing and using your oils

In this chapter you will learn:
- *how to recognize high-quality pure essential oils*
- *how to care for and store your oils*
- *some of the many different ways of using essential oils.*

Quality and adulteration

It is vital to use only high-quality pure essential oils for optimum results. It is most unfortunate that many essential oils available on the market today are of poor quality and, therefore, cannot help alleviate health problems. Only five per cent of all essential oils produced in the world are used for aromatherapy. Essential oil traders supply mostly to the perfume, food, pharmaceutical and chemical manufacturing industries. The food and perfume industries are more concerned with the fragrance or flavour of an oil rather than its therapeutic effects. These industries must always have essential oils with the same chemical formulae if they are to produce the same aroma and taste consistently, so they find it necessary to 'adulterate' oils to replicate aromas and flavours. Price is also a major consideration. Factors such as the weather, bad harvests, the variety of the plant, the composition of the soil, the time and the method of cultivation and extraction can affect the composition of essential oils greatly and this creates difficulties for the perfume and food industries who seek standardization.

Suppliers of essential oils will sometimes adulterate their oils by adding synthetic ingredients, alcohols, vegetable oil, cheap chemical constituents or low-cost essential oils. They may even substitute an entire essential oil with a cheaper, similar oil for commercial gain (e.g. lavendin may be sold as lavender).

Essential oils used in aromatherapy must, of course, be as pure, natural and 'whole' as possible if they are to have the desired therapeutic effects. Synthetic materials which simulate the aroma and appearance of an essential oil cannot have the same therapeutic properties as an essential oil and should not be used in therapy. Synthetic chemicals also carry the risk of harmful and unpleasant side-effects, as do synthetic drugs. If oils are referred to as 'nature identical' this implies that the oil is synthetic and produced in the laboratory and is, therefore, unsuitable for aromatherapy. Synthetic oils also do not possess the 'vital force' or 'life force' of essential oils which comes from living plants. Nor do chemicals contain the 'vibration' of natural living plants.

Insight

It is totally impossible to duplicate an essential oil in its entirety in the laboratory. Vital constituents and trace elements will inevitably be missing. It is the *total* of the components of an essential oil working together which produces a healing effect.

Since most aromatherapy suppliers buy essential oils from importers who supply the perfume and food industries it is important to seek a supplier who deals mainly with essential oils intended only for therapeutic use. I have found over the years that purchasing essential oils is a matter of trust. (See Taking it further for information regarding suppliers.)

Care and storage

Essential oils are extremely precious and should be treated with respect – they can also be very expensive. They are damaged by ultraviolet light and deteriorate more rapidly at the blue end of the spectrum than the red. Therefore, essential oils should be stored in amber-coloured bottles (if you do keep your essential oils in blue bottles then they should be kept in the dark – this is less important if your bottles are brown).

Insight
Never buy essential oils stored in clear glass or plastic bottles or decant them into such bottles. They should never be placed in direct sunlight. Remember that amber-coloured bottles are most effective for storing essential oils.

Essential oils should never be placed in direct sunlight so avoid sunny windowsills or shelves on radiators – no matter how attractive the bottles look! Essential oils do not like extremes of temperatures. They are highly volatile, which means that they evaporate rapidly. Always replace the caps immediately and ensure that the tops are tightly closed when the oils are not in use. Essential oils must be cared for properly to prevent chemical degradation (i.e. a process whereby the quality of the essential oil is reduced over time) which will occur with prolonged storage and poor storage conditions.

Pure essential oils will last for approximately three years from the bottling date. In excellent storage conditions (i.e. amber bottles in a cool place with no air space) they will keep for about five years. Citrus oils tend to have a shorter shelf life due to their high proportion of terpenes, as do absolutes and resins; these thicken even more with age and the smell of the solvent becomes more noticeable.

Once essential oils have been diluted in a carrier oil, the shelf life reduces dramatically. For maximum benefit use freshly made-up blends. A blend will keep for about three to six months if it is stored in an amber-coloured bottle in a cool place away from sunlight. If wheatgerm oil is added then the shelf life is approximately six to nine months. If the smell alters and the vegetable oil becomes rancid then you should definitely discard it.

Dos and don'ts of buying and storage

▶ *Clear glass or plastic bottles do not contain pure essential oils. Always buy oils in amber-coloured bottles.*

▶ *How old are the essential oils? When were they bottled?*

▶ *Are the oils in direct sunlight?*

▶ *Are the essential oils all the same price? If they are, then you are definitely not purchasing pure essential oils. For instance, pure essential oil of rose will be far more expensive than lavender or rosemary.*

▶ *Have the essential oils been diluted with any carrier oils? If so, when were they blended?*

▶ *Have the essential oils been adulterated with synthetic materials or bulking agents?*

▶ *Does the aromatherapy trader deal mostly with the perfume and food industries? Always look for an aromatherapy specialist.*

▶ *Does your supplier know about the essential oils?*

▶ *If blends are being sold, is there a qualified aromatherapist on the staff?*

▶ *Has the supplier been recommended to you?*

▶ *How long has the aromatherapy firm been established?*

▶ *Essential oils should always be kept away from young children. If they are taken internally some essential oils can be highly dangerous.*

▶ *Never leave bottled pure essential oils standing on plastic, polished or painted surfaces which can be damaged by the chemical constituents.*

▶ *Always store essential oils away from naked flames.*

▶ *Store essential oils away from your homoeopathic medications which may be antidoted by the more powerful aromas.*

Insight

Two tips for checking for the purity of essential oils:

1 Put one drop of pure essential oil on a piece of paper and see if it leaves a greasy mark. If your essential oil is pure

then there should be no greasy mark. Despite their name essential oils are not oily.

2 Rub a little essential oil between your thumb and index finger. Does it have a greasy feel? If it does then the oil has been adulterated.

Using essential oils

There are numerous ways in which essential oils can be used. I will outline some of the easiest and most effective techniques, but I urge you to be creative and fill your home with essential oils. You can create a beautiful aromatic environment while preventing or healing a multitude of common disorders.

EXTERNAL USE

Baths
Aromatherapy baths have been employed for pleasure and therapeutic purposes throughout history. The Greek physician Hippocrates, the Father of Medicine, claimed that 'the way to health is to have an aromatic bath and a scented massage daily'.

Baths were particularly enjoyed by the ancient Egyptians, who had public baths, as did the Romans, for whom baths were an important aspect of social life. Water itself is therapeutic: 'water cures' are advocated by naturopaths, and various forms of hydrotherapy can be found in use nowadays at health farms and natural therapy centres. Baths are an effective way of using essential oils as the oils act in two ways: by absorption into the skin and by inhalation.

Essential oils are simple to use in the bath. Just fill the bath and sprinkle about six drops of your chosen undiluted oil into the water, agitating it thoroughly. Do not add the essential oil until you have run the bath completely, otherwise the oil will evaporate with the heat of the water and the therapeutic properties will be lost before you climb in! Always disperse the oil – if you inadvertently sit down on neat essential oil of, say, tangerine you will jump up again very quickly! Shut the door to keep the precious aromas in and stay in the bath for at least 15 minutes to allow the oil to penetrate deeply into your body tissues.

> ## Insight
>
> Remember to use just six drops of essential oil in your bath. To de-stress try two drops of geranium, two drops lavender and two drops ylang ylang. To wake you up or to rejuvenate after a long hard day try two drops of rosemary, two drops lemon and two drops black pepper.

As essential oils are not soluble in water you may blend your six drops of essential oil with a teaspoon of carrier oil for a moisturizing bath. This is particularly beneficial for those with dry skin, although carrier oils can leave a greasy ring around the bath. However, special, unscented bath oils, which contain natural dispersing agents, can be purchased. These leave the skin feeling soft but not greasy. Choose any vegetable oil such as sweet almond, wheatgerm, avocado or jojoba. You could mix up enough oil for several baths. Your skin will feel soft, nourished and supple.

Absolutes and resinoids such as jasmine and benzoin should be blended with a teaspoon of carrier oil as they tend to sink to the bottom of the bath and are difficult to clean off! I would strongly advise anyone with a sensitive skin to *always* blend the essential oil with a carrier oil. Also, when using essential oils in a bath for babies and young children the oils should always be blended with a carrier oil. Undiluted essential oils can damage the eyes and babies and toddlers do have a tendency to rub their eyes.

Use one drop in a baby's bath and two drops in a toddler's bath diluted in a teaspoon of a carrier oil such as sweet almond oil. I can endorse the effectiveness of this method.

Any essential oil may be added to a bath. Although caution should be exercised with the citrus oils and the stronger essences such as black pepper and peppermint if you have particularly sensitive skin. Just add three drops instead of six.

Essential oils may also be added to sea salt or magnesium sulphate. Bath salts help to promote detoxification and also relieve aching muscles. To make your own aromatherapy bath salts add no more than 1 ml of essential oils to 100 g of salt.

Hydrotherapy baths and Jacuzzis
Use the same number of drops as you would in a normal bath, although if it is a large hydrotherapy bath designed for two to three persons then ten drops may be added. Sprinkle in your essential oils after the bath has been filled. The essential oils must not be diluted in vegetable oils, which can coat the pipes.

Footbaths and hand baths
Footbaths and hand baths are highly beneficial in situations where it is impractical to enjoy a full aromatherapy bath – perhaps if you are elderly or have a disability. Footbaths, in particular, are incredibly relaxing at the end of a long, hard day especially when you feel too lethargic to undress. They are excellent for foot conditions such as athlete's foot and pain and swelling in the feet. Hand baths help to relieve the pain, stiffness and swelling of arthritis. Anyone who uses their hands extensively, such as hairdressers, gardeners or those working with computers, should have regular hand baths.

Add six drops of essential oil to a bowl of hand-hot water just before you immerse your feet or hands and soak for about ten to fifteen minutes. If you wish you may mix your essential oils with a carrier oil.

Insight
There is no excuse for not having time for aromatherapy. Enjoy a footbath while you are reading or studying and a hand or footbath while watching your favourite television programme. Remember to use six drops.

Sitz baths and bidets
A sitz bath is beneficial in cases of cystitis, haemorrhoids, vaginal discharge, stitches after childbirth and so on. Sprinkle about four to

six drops of pure essential oil into a bowl of hand-hot water and sit in the bowl for about ten minutes. Your essential oils may be added to a carrier oil. If you have a bidet then use the same number of drops. Ensure that the essential oil and water are thoroughly mixed.

Jug douche
This method is excellent for combating vaginal discharge and infections as well as anal problems. Boil a kettle and allow the water to cool in a one-litre jug ensuring that there is no limescale. Add six drops of essential oil. Lift both the seat and the lid of the toilet. Stand over the toilet and pour the solution over the vaginal and anal area. Dry the area gently.

If you wish to carry out this treatment at work you can prepare the solution in a one-litre plastic bottle.

Showers
A shower can never be as relaxing as a bath when using essential oils. However, it can be quite a stimulating way to begin your day.

Apply six drops of essential oil to a sponge or a flannel and rub all over your body towards the end of your shower. Alternatively, add six drops of essential oil to two teaspoons of carrier oil and apply to your body before stepping into the shower. Make sure that you inhale the warming vapours. Another method is to plug the tray of your shower, turn on the water and add six drops of essential oil to the water. You will absorb the oils through your feet and as the vapours rise you will inhale them.

Some essential oil suppliers stock shower gel to which essential oils may be added. (See Taking it further for information regarding suppliers.)

Compresses
Compresses can be used for a variety of disorders such as muscular aches and pains, bruises, rheumatic and arthritic pain, headaches and sprains. They are a very effective way of relieving pain and reducing inflammation and swelling.

You may apply compresses either hot or cold. Alternate hot and cold compresses are valuable for treating sprains. As a general rule, where there is fever, acute pain or hot swellings use a cold compress. When treating chronic (long-term) pain use a hot compress.

To make a compress, mix approximately six drops of essential oil into a small bowl of hot or cold water. Soak any piece of absorbent material such as a flannel, handkerchief, piece of sheeting or towelling in the solution ensuring that as much essential oil as possible is absorbed by your fabric. Squeeze out the compress so it does not drip everywhere and apply to the affected area. Wrap clingfilm around it or secure with a bandage. Leave for about two hours or even overnight. Where there is a fever replace with a new cold compress when necessary.

Insight
Two tips!

1 Apply a lavender compress to your forehead or the back of your neck to relieve a fever or a headache.
2 Make a compress using two drops lavender, two drops peppermint and two drops rosemary. Place on the affected area to relieve muscular aches and joint pain.

Gargles and mouthwashes
Gargles are particularly beneficial for sore throats, respiratory problems, loss of voice and halitosis (bad breath). After dental surgery gargling can help to relieve pains and inflammation, reduce blood flow and speed up the healing process. Gargle twice daily, although if the problem is acute then you can gargle every two hours.

Put two drops of essential oil into half a glass of water. Stir well, gargle and spit it out. Do not swallow. Stir again and repeat. You may also use one to two teaspoons of organic cider vinegar or lemon and/or a teaspoon of honey in your gargle. Honey has anti-inflammatory and antibacterial properties and is renowned for its soothing action on the throat, and fresh lemon juice is antibacterial, detoxifying and counteracts acidity. Antiseptic oils such as tea tree, lemon and thyme are excellent for treating sore throats. German/Roman chamomile, geranium and sandalwood will also soothe inflammation. Myrrh and tea tree combined is very useful for treating mouth ulcers.

INHALATIONS

Inhalation of essential oils works upon the body, mind and spirit.

On a physical level there is a strong action on the mucous membranes of the nose, the lungs and the respiratory system in general. Conditions such as asthma, bronchitis, catarrh, coughs, colds, sinusitis and sore throats can all benefit enormously.

The inhalation of essential oils has a profound effect on the nervous system, helping to relieve insomnia, anxiety and stress-related disorders and lifting depression and negativity.

On a spiritual level some essential oils such as frankincense, cedarwood and linden blossom raise the consciousness and provide an excellent aid for meditation.

Steam inhalation

Add three drops of essential oil to a bowl of hot water. Cover your head with a towel and lean over the bowl inhaling deeply for a few minutes. Keep your eyes closed to avoid irritation. If someone who has asthma uses this method then just one drop is adequate. Take care with the hot water if there are small children around.

Insight

One of my favourite oils as an inhalation for catarrh and sinusitis is essential oil of cajeput. Try it next time you have a cold to loosen up mucus and speed up your recovery.

Water bowl

Put boiling water into a small bowl and add two to six drops of essential oil. Place the bowl in a warm place, if possible, for maximum effect (e.g. on a radiator). Ensure that small children do not drink the solution or knock it over. Close the doors and windows for a few minutes to enable the aroma to fill the room.

Handkerchief/tissue
Sprinkle a few drops of essential oil on to a handkerchief, paper towel or tissue and take a few deep breaths. This method is particularly effective for relieving nasal congestion (use cajeput, eucalyptus) and also for stopping panic attacks (use lavender). Place the handkerchief in your pocket and you can continue to inhale the aroma throughout the day. Sufferers of motion sickness will also find this method effective.

Hands
In a crisis situation put one drop of lavender on to your palm, rub your hands together, cup them over your nose and then breathe deeply. Avoid the eye area and ensure that your eyes are closed.

It is not a good idea to open a bottle of essential oil and inhale straight from it. Frequent opening of essential oils accelerates the rate of evaporation and therapeutic properties are lost. Also, removing essential oils stains from your carpet can be expensive!

Room spray
A room spray is an excellent way of purifying the atmosphere. Pour 250 ml of water into a plant spray and add 15–20 drops of essential oil. Shake the bottle well and spray the room. You can even spray carpets and curtains. Do not spray on to polished surfaces.

Sprays can also be used to relieve irritation and pain as in chickenpox, shingles, burns and any infectious skin diseases.

Vaporizers and diffusers
Electric vaporizers are sometimes used in clinics and hospital settings since they are considered to be safe. Electric diffusers, which do not use heat, are also becoming popular. However, both vaporizers and diffusers particularly can be rather expensive.

It is also very important to use exact and small doses – essential oils can be harmful and even dangerous in high doses. A safe dose is just two to three drops of essential oil to be taken three times a day. After three weeks stop taking the essential oils internally in order to rest the body and enable the liver to eliminate any toxic overload. As essential oils taste so powerful and bitter and can cause irritation they should be ingested in one of the following ways:

2–3 drops in a little red wine

or

2–3 drops in honey water (one teaspoon of honey to one-third cup of water) or in a spoonful of honey

or

2–3 drops in a dessertspoon of olive oil (extra virgin)

or

2–3 drops on a sugar lump

Take three times daily for no more than three weeks.

Aromatherapists do not prescribe essential oils for internal use, as their insurance does not cover internal use. However, many have used the above method effectively, with no side effects, for a long time. It is particularly good for treating sore throats and other respiratory problems, as well as for digestive problems such as indigestion and constipation, and urinary disorders such as cystitis.

Do not give essential oils by mouth to babies or pregnant women.

TEST YOUR KNOWLEDGE

1 *What colour bottles should essential oils be stored in?*

2 *Are all essential oils approximately the same price?*

3 *How many drops of essential oil are used for the following methods?*
   a *bath/shower*
   b *footbath/hand bath*
   c *compress*
   d *gargle*

4 *How many drops of essential oil do you use to each 10 ml of carrier oil?*

4

Carrier/base/fixed oils

In this chapter you will learn:
* *the therapeutic properties and uses of a wide range of carrier oils recommended for use in aromatherapy.*

Essential oils are highly concentrated in their pure state and they should not be used undiluted directly on the skin. Therefore, a natural medium is required for an aromatherapy massage treatment and is referred to as the carrier, base or fixed oil. Since the carrier oil constitutes a large proportion of an aromatherapy blend its quality should be given careful consideration. Carrier oils as well as essential oils should be of the highest quality if maximum therapeutic benefits are to be obtained.

The carrier oil chosen should be cold pressed. In the process of cold pressing the use of excessive heat is avoided and therefore any changes to the natural characteristics of the oil are minimized. Oils produced by the process of 'hot extraction', although much cheaper, are unsuitable for use in aromatherapy as they are of an inferior quality.

The base oil should also be unrefined and untreated by chemicals. The process of refining includes the removal of colour by bleaching, removing taste and smell, extracting natural fatty acids, which can lead to cloudiness, and the removal of free fatty acids.

Vegetable oils have therapeutic properties in their own right and contain many vitamins and minerals, but the more highly processed the vegetable oils are, the less vitamin content will be retained. Colour, other additives and synthetic antioxidants to extend the shelf life may also be added at the oil pressing factories, which is also undesirable. For the purpose of aromatherapy always use cold pressed (preferably the 'virgin' type which is the first oil to be collected), unrefined, additive-free carrier oils. It is highly unlikely that you will find these oils on the shelves of your supermarket! Since the carrier oil is by far the largest part of any massage blend, always choose it carefully.

Mineral oil (purified, light petroleum oil), such as commercial baby oil, should never be used in aromatherapy as a carrier oil. Mineral oils tend to clog the pores whereas some of the vegetable oil molecules are absorbed through the skin. Mineral oils also do not have the nutritional constituents (vitamins, minerals and fatty acids) of the vegetable oils which nourish and benefit the skin. Mineral oil is used by the cosmetics industry because it does not become rancid. However, it stays on the skin like an 'oil slick' and prevents it from breathing.

The shelf life of a base oil is dependent upon its fatty acid and vitamin E content. Vegetable oils which have a high proportion of saturated fatty acids will keep longer than those which are high in unsaturated fatty acids. The presence of vitamin E in the carrier oil will also increase the shelf life.

There is a wide variety of vegetable oils suitable for aromatherapy massage. Some of the most commonly used carrier oils include sweet almond, apricot kernel, peach kernel and grapeseed. These oils are not too thick and have hardly any smell and so will not mask the aroma of the essential oils. Some aromatherapists will use these carrier oils on their own but many prefer to add other thicker, more viscous oils to their aromatherapy blends, such as avocado, jojoba and evening primrose oil. My own particular special blend includes sweet almond, apricot and peach kernel, jojoba, avocado, calendula and wheatgerm.

Insight

When choosing a carrier oil factors to bear in mind include:

▶ *quality (choose a cold-pressed, unrefined, additive-free oil)*
▶ *texture (thick, sticky oils do NOT make a good massage medium)*
▶ *absorbability (choose a vegetable and NOT a mineral oil)*
▶ *aroma (a strong smell will mask the aroma of the essential oils).*

The following section lists and describes the principal properties and indications of a wide range of carrier oils. Please note that some carrier oils are used on their own, or they may be blended with the thicker, more viscous carrier oils.

ALMOND OIL (SWEET)

Latin name: *Prunus amygdalis* var. *dulcis*

Family: *Rosaceae*

Sweet almond oil is one of the most widely used carrier oils in aromatherapy since it is low in odour and is not too thick, sticky or heavy. It is easily absorbed by the skin and is highly recommended for aromamassage (see Chapter 7).

The almond tree is an ancient tree that has been cultivated for thousands of years and was highly prized by the Greeks who brought almonds to Southern Europe. The fruits of the almond tree look like a small green apricot and the best quality oil, which is extracted by cold pressing the kernels, is pale yellow in colour. It has a delicate, rather sweet smell and is rich in vitamins and unsaturated fatty acids. If the oil is refined and chemically extracted it is cheaper due to the higher yield but such oil is not really suitable for aromatherapy.

Uses:
▶ *beneficial for all skin types*
▶ *an excellent emollient for nourishing the skin*

- *helps to relieve itching induced by conditions such as eczema, psoriasis and dermatitis*
- *soothes inflammation*
- *nourishes dry and prematurely aged skin*
- *suitable for sensitive skin*
- *soothes sunburn*
- *excellent for moisturizing dry hair that has been chemically treated or exposed to too much sun.*

Sweet almond oil is highly recommended and may be used as a base oil up to 100 per cent.

Special precautions:
Sweet almond oil is considered to be a very safe carrier oil. There is an essential oil of bitter almond which is toxic and is never used in aromatherapy due to the risk of the formation of prussic acid during extraction.

APRICOT KERNEL OIL

Latin name: *Prunus armeniaca*

Family: *Rosaceae*

Apricot kernel oil is very similar to sweet almond oil although it is more expensive as it is produced in smaller quantities.

The tree originated in China (apricot kernels are used in traditional Chinese medicine) and was brought to the Middle East and then by the Romans to Southern Europe. The oil is obtained by cold pressing the kernels and contains vitamins and unsaturated fatty acids.

Insight
Apricot kernel oil is used in many cosmetic products, such as in facial scrubs and masks, to clear away dead skin cells, as well as in soaps, shampoos and creams.

The oil is pale yellow and has a stronger odour than sweet almond – rather marzipan-like. Apricot kernel oil has a wonderful silky texture and is easily absorbed by the skin. It is a most delightful carrier oil to use in an aromamassage.

Uses:
- ▶ *excellent for all skin types*
- ▶ *nourishes dry skin*
- ▶ *relieves itching and therefore helps conditions such as eczema*
- ▶ *beneficial for sensitive and prematurely aged skin.*

Apricot kernel oil may be used as a base 100 per cent although it is usually added to a blend due to its enriching and nourishing properties. It is an excellent choice for a facial oil.

Special precautions:
Apricot kernel oil is completely safe with no reported toxic effects. Interestingly, however, ingestion of apricot kernels is the most common form of cyanide poison – so avoid eating them!

Insight

Four of the most commonly used carrier oils for aromatherapy are sweet almond, apricot kernel, peach kernel and grapeseed, as these oils are not thick. They have hardly any odour and therefore will not mask the aroma of your essential oil(s).

They can be used on their own or blended with small amounts of the thicker, more viscous oils such as avocado and jojoba.

For example, combine 80% sweet almond and 5% each of avocado, calendula, jojoba and wheatgerm.

AVOCADO OIL

Latin name: *Persea americana*

Family: *Lauraceae*

The avocado tree originates from the tropical and sub-tropical areas of the Americas. The Spaniards discovered it there in the fifteenth century and then brought it to Europe.

This wonderful dark rich green carrier oil is cold pressed from the dried flesh of avocado pears which have been damaged and therefore are not of a high enough quality for marketing. True cold-pressed avocado oil is not very common and therefore the refined oil, which is a pale yellow colour, is usually sold. However, the unrefined, cold-pressed oil is the one to use. If the oil is slightly cloudy in cold conditions, if there is a deposit present, and if the oil is a rich green colour then this indicates it has not been through an extensive refining process. Avocado is used in many cosmetic preparations including lipsticks, creams, lotions and shampoos.

Insight

The flesh of an avocado pear may be crushed and applied to the skin to counteract dryness after a holiday in the sun, although avocado oil is far less messy!

It also has a distinctive aroma similar to the ripe fruit. Avocado oil is rich in lecithin, vitamins A, B and D and minerals as well as saturated and unsaturated fatty acids. It has a long shelf life.

Uses:

- *moisturizes and softens all types of skin*
- *beneficial for dry, dehydrated skin as it is such a highly penetrative oil*
- *soothes skin inflammation*
- *prevents premature ageing*
- *helps to heal the skin*
- *may help poor circulation*
- *maintains the suppleness and elasticity of the skin*
- *offers some protection from the sun and is sometimes mixed with sesame oil for this purpose.*

Avocado oil is usually added to a blend in up to a 10 per cent dilution.

Special precautions:
A very safe oil which does not cause sensitization, but do not use the colourless, refined, bleached oil.

BORAGE OIL

Latin name: *Borago officinalis*

Family: *Boraginaceae*

Borage originated from the Middle East but is now a widely grown herb. It is sometimes known as 'beebread' since bees are attracted to it. The ancients believed that borage was a plant that brought happiness to the melancholic.

To obtain the oil, the dark brown borage seeds are cold pressed. Borage oil is an extremely rich source of the essential fatty acid GLA (gamma linolenic acid) – it contains 16–23 per cent as compared with evening primrose oil which contains approximately nine per cent. Borage oil has almost no odour and therefore will not mask essential oils in an aromatherapy blend. It is an excellent addition to a facial oil.

Uses:
- *highly recommended for premature ageing*
- *prevents wrinkles*
- *nourishes dry and dehydrated skin*
- *soothes itching in conditions such as eczema and psoriasis*
- *ideal for dry, coloured or permed hair.*

Borage oil is usually added to a blend in up to a 10 per cent dilution.

Special precautions:
Borage oil is very safe with no known contraindications.

CALENDULA OIL (ALSO KNOWN AS MARIGOLD OIL)

Latin name: *Calendula officinalis*

Family: *Asteraceae* (or *Compositae*)

Calendula oil is a macerated oil which means that the wonderful yellow or bright orange flowers are macerated in a fixed oil to produce the orange-yellow coloured calendula oil. The plant has its origins in the Mediterranean area and it has been cultivated since the Middle Ages. It is highly valued by herbalists, and infusions, extracts and tinctures have been very popular remedies. Calendula oil should not be confused with the essential oil Tagetes which is also often referred to as marigold.

Uses:
- ▶ *renowned for all skin disorders*
- ▶ *soothes inflammation*
- ▶ *heals chapped and cracked skin*
- ▶ *useful for varicose veins and broken veins*
- ▶ *relieves itching and skin conditions such as eczema*
- ▶ *helps to reduce thread veins on the face*
- ▶ *soothes and heals cracked nipples*
- ▶ *reduces and prevents scarring*
- ▶ *useful for bruises*
- ▶ *soothes burns*
- ▶ *makes a wonderful addition to hand and foot creams.*

Calendula oil would normally be added to your basic carrier oil in up to a 10 per cent dilution, although it may be used in its own right on specific areas.

Special precautions:
Calendula oil has no known side-effects.

CARROT OIL/WILD CARROT OIL

Latin name: *Daucus carota*

Family: *Apiaceae* (or *Umbelliferae*)

Carrot oil is a macerated oil which is prepared by finely chopping up the carrot and leaving it to steep in a vegetable oil. The chosen vegetable oil is usually sunflower and the mixture is macerated for about three weeks and then filtered to produce the carrot oil. It is rich in beta-carotene as well as vitamins A, B, C, D, E and F. The oil is a clear orange liquid.

Carrot oil should not be confused with the essential oil of carrot which should never be used undiluted as a base oil.

Uses:
- ▶ *soothes itchy skin*
- ▶ *helpful for psoriasis and eczema*
- ▶ *highly recommended for mature skin*
- ▶ *may help to prevent wrinkles*
- ▶ *assists the healing process of skin*
- ▶ *beneficial for dry skin.*

Carrot oil would not usually be used on its own 100 per cent but is added in up to a 10 per cent dilution.

Special precautions:
Carrot oil has no contraindications.

COCONUT OIL

Latin name: *Cocos nucifera*

Family: *Palmae*

The palm tree is believed to have originated in the Indian Ocean region. The coconut is now grown in many tropical areas due to its commercial importance. Interestingly 'cocos' is the Portuguese word for monkey as the nut resembles a monkey's face!

Coconut oil is usually solvent extracted and is primarily composed of saturated fatty acids. It is used a great deal in India in Ayurvedic medicine for a variety of complaints. Coconut oil is widely used in Southern India as it is thought to keep the head cool. It is one of the most popular oils employed for Indian head massage. (See *Teach Yourself Indian Head Massage*) Many soap formulations and hair conditioners contain coconut oil because of its moisturizing properties. Coconut oil is not used a great deal in aromatherapy treatments.

Uses:
▶ *beneficial for dry and chapped skin*
▶ *excellent for dry, brittle or chemically treated hair.*

Special precautions:
Care should be taken with hypersensitive skin as in rare cases it has been known to cause skin rashes.

EVENING PRIMROSE OIL

Latin name: *Oenorthera biennis*

Family: *Onagraceae*

The plant is native to North America and was introduced into Europe in the seventeenth century. The oil is cold pressed from the seeds and is rich in linoleic acid (approximately 70 per cent), which is in a polyunsaturated fatty acid, and also contains GLA (gamma linoleic acid), which is also present in borage oil.

Insight
Heralded as a 'miracle of modern times' it has become increasingly popular to take evening primrose oil internally in capsules for a whole host of conditions including:

(Contd)

- *prevention of heart disease*
- *lowering of blood cholesterol and blood pressure*
- *premenstrual syndrome (PMS), menopause and other menstrual irregularities*
- *skin conditions such as eczema and psoriasis*
- *allergic conditions*
- *asthma and hayfever*
- *mental disorders such as hyperactivity in children and schizophrenia*
- *multiple sclerosis*
- *diabetes*
- *Raynaud's disease.*

Uses:
- *excellent for dry skin*
- *ideal for sensitive and allergic-type skin*
- *calms down redness and inflammation*
- *counteracts premature ageing of the skin and wrinkles*
- *favourable for skin conditions aggravated by hormonal imbalances, e.g. acne and puberty, prior to menstruation and during the menopause*
- *may improve varicose veins*
- *beneficial for dry hair and dandruff.*

Evening primrose oil is usually added to a blend in up to a 10 per cent dilution.

Special precautions:
Evening primrose oil is a very safe oil when used externally.

GRAPESEED OIL

Latin name: *Vitis vinifera*

Family: *Vitaceae*

Grapeseed oil was first produced in France and now comes mainly from Italy, Spain and California.

It is produced by hot extraction which is necessary since there is only about 12 per cent oil in the seeds. The extracted oil may then be refined. Unfortunately it is not available cold pressed (and cold-pressed, unrefined oils are the finest oils for aromatherapy). However, it is a very popular oil for massage and aromatherapy as it is a very smooth oil which is not greasy and is also colourless and odourless. It contains a high percentage of linoleic acid and also vitamin E.

Uses:
▶ *may be used on all skin types*
▶ *easily absorbed by the skin.*

Grapeseed oil can be used as a base oil 100 per cent.

Special precautions:
It is a very safe oil with no known contraindications.

JOJOBA OIL

Latin name: *Simmondsia chinensis/Simmondsia sinensis*

Family: *Buxaceae*

This plant grows in the desert regions of Southern California, Arizona and Northwest Mexico. It can be planted to save arid land from becoming desert.

Jojoba is not really an oil but is rather a liquid wax. It is extracted from the crushed seeds and is made up of esters formed from long chain fatty acids and long chain fatty alcohols. Another constituent is myristic acid which is an anti-inflammatory agent. The oil was discovered to have the same properties as sperm whale oil and has taken its place in the cosmetics industry since the whale became an endangered species.

It is a golden oil which is very stable and as it does not oxidize it does not become rancid and has a very long shelf life. If jojoba oil is left in a very cold place it will solidify, but will very rapidly liquefy when brought back to room temperature. It has a faint, slightly sweet aroma and a wonderful texture. Jojoba is used in creams, lotions and lipsticks.

Uses:
- ▶ *combats inflammation and therefore is useful for arthritis, dermatitis and swellings of all descriptions*
- ▶ *suitable for all types of skin*
- ▶ *nourishes and moisturizes dry skin*
- ▶ *combats the drying effects of the sun*
- ▶ *helps to heal wounds*
- ▶ *beneficial for chapped skin and nappy rash*
- ▶ *prevents the build-up of sebum and therefore useful for oily skin*
- ▶ *relieves itchy skin conditions such as eczema and psoriasis*
- ▶ *helps control acne*
- ▶ *conditions, protects and renews the hair.*

Jojoba is usually added in up to a 10 per cent dilution as it is more expensive than some other base oils. However, it may be used 100 per cent on small areas.

Insight

Jojoba makes a wonderful facial oil which can be compared favourably with any expensive cream.

Blend jojoba with essential oils such as rose, frankincense, neroli and carrot seed to prevent and reduce the signs of ageing.

Special precautions:
A safe carrier oil which I have never seen any reactions to but allergic reactions have been rarely reported.

OLIVE OIL

Latin name: *Olea europaea*

Family: *Oleaceae*

The olive tree has been cultivated and used for thousands of years. The olive branch has long been regarded as a token of peace and olive leaf garlands were worn by the Greeks. Olive trees do not begin to produce fruit until after 15 years, but they can live for hundreds of years.

Olive oil (like avocado oil) is extracted from the flesh of the fruit. After the fruit has been pressed the resulting oil is filtered and the first portion of the oil is known as 'virgin' oil with the oil obtained at the beginning of the pressing being known as 'extra virgin'. It contains oleic acid and unsaturated fatty acids including linoleic acid.

Olive oil is slightly green due to a small amount of chlorophyll from the flesh. It should have a distinctive, slightly fruity aroma if it is of a high quality and suitable for use in aromatherapy. The ability of olive oil taken in the diet to lower the blood pressure and protect against heart disease is well known. It is also beneficial for the liver and the stomach and it has a laxative effect.

Uses:
- *useful for dry skin and scalp*
- *relieves itching of the skin*
- *combats inflammation and may reduce swellings*
- *combats dry, damaged, brittle hair*
- *used in detox regimes (see* Teach Yourself Detox*)*
- *alleviates muscular aches and pains*
- *helps reduce bruises*
- *may prevent wrinkles*
- *affords some protection from the sun and is sometimes blended with sesame and avocado for this purpose.*

Olive oil is not usually used 100 per cent as it is too heavy for massage and if used is usually added in up to a 10 per cent dilution.

Special precautions:
Olive oil is a very safe carrier oil provided an excellent quality oil is used.

PEACH KERNEL OIL

Latin name: *Prunus persica*

Family: *Rosaceae*

The peach tree originates from China. The Romans brought the peach to Europe. It was introduced to America in the seventeenth century and California and Texas are now the world's major producers.

Peach kernel oil is very similar to apricot kernel oil and sweet almond oil. It is extracted by cold pressing the kernels if it is a high quality oil and is made up mostly of unsaturated fatty acids including linoleic acid. It is pale yellow in colour and virtually odourless with a light texture which makes it a wonderful carrier oil for aromatherapy.

Uses:
- *an effective moisturizer for dry, dehydrated skin*
- *relieves itching as in eczema and psoriasis*
- *beneficial for mature skin*
- *suitable for dry, damaged or coloured hair*
- *good for sensitive skin.*

Peach kernel oil may be used as a base 100 per cent although it is usually added to a blend in a dilution of approximately 10 per cent.

Special precautions:
Peach kernel oil is totally safe with no reported side-effects.

SESAME OIL

Latin name: *Sesamum indicum*

Family: *Pedaliaceae*

The sesame plant originated from the tropical regions of the East Indies but is now grown worldwide. It has been cultivated and was highly regarded by the ancients for thousands of years – it was one of the plants placed in Tutankhamen's tomb.

In ancient Egypt the seeds were ground to produce a flour and today they are widely ground into the well-known paste 'tahini'. If sesame and honey are mixed together the result is the delicious 'halva' which the women of ancient Babylon believed helped them to retain both their beauty and their youth.

The oil is obtained by cold pressing the seeds which contain up to 55 per cent oil. It should be a clear pale yellow colour as the bleached sesame oil is not suitable for aromatherapy. Sesame oil is almost odourless which again makes it acceptable as a carrier oil. The oil is rich in vitamins A, B and E as well as in minerals such as calcium and phosphorus – vitamin E gives the oil excellent keeping qualities.

Insight

Sesame oil is a popular oil in India and is used extensively in Ayurvedic medicine. It is a must-have oil for Indian head massage. It is also thought to prevent the hair from turning grey.

Uses:
- *beneficial for all types of skin*
- *recommended for dry, dehydrated skin*
- *prevents ageing*
- *combats muscular aches and pains*
- *reduces swelling*
- *helpful for skin conditions such as eczema and psoriasis*
- *may reduce broken veins*
- *prevents greyness and restores hair colour*
- *provides some sun protection and may be blended with olive and avocado.*

Sesame oil may be used 100 per cent but it is usually added to a carrier oil.

Special precautions:
Reaction is very unlikely to occur but take care with highly
sensitive skin.

WHEATGERM OIL

Latin name: *Triticum vulgare*

Family: *Graminae*

This plant is native to West Asia and the oil is extracted from the
germ. The wheatgerm is stirred into a high-quality, cold-pressed
oil so that the oil is soaked up by the germ. Cold pressing is then
performed to yield an oil composed of one third wheatgerm oil
and two thirds base oil (e.g. sweet almond, olive, etc.).

Wheatgerm oil is well known for containing high levels of
vitamin E which is a natural antioxidant which may be added as
a preservative. It also contains vitamins A and B as well as many
minerals including zinc, iron, potassium, sulphur and magnesium.
The unsaturated fatty acid linoleic acid is also present.

Wheatgerm oil is a rich orangey-brown colour with a strong
odour.

Uses:
- ▶ *nourishes dry and cracked skin*
- ▶ *revitalizes mature skin – its natural antioxidants fight free radicals*
- ▶ *relieves itchy skin conditions such as eczema, dermatitis and psoriasis*
- ▶ *useful for anti-ageing*
- ▶ *prevents and reduces stretch marks and scars*
- ▶ *beneficial for dry and brittle hair.*

Wheatgerm oil is heavy and has a strong odour and therefore
would not be used on its own. It is usually added in up to a
10 per cent dilution to preserve the life of a blend.

Special precautions:
Take care with individuals who have a wheat allergy. If you wish, test a small area of the skin for a skin reaction prior to an aromatherapy treatment or simply avoid using it.

Other carrier oils

The oils I have already described are among the most popular used in aromatherapy.

However, there are a number of other carrier oils that may be used, according to personal preference, and I will describe these in brief.

HAZELNUT OIL

Latin name: *Corylus avellana*

Family name: *Corylaceae*

An amber-yellow oil obtained by cold pressing and then filtering. It has a distinctive aroma.

Uses:
- ▶ *moisturizes the skin*
- ▶ *beneficial for oily skins, acne and combination skins*
- ▶ *helpful for poor circulation*
- ▶ *provides some protection against the sun.*

Special precautions:
Take care with allergic individuals.

KUKUI NUT OIL

Latin name: *Aleurites moluccana*

Family name: *Euphorbiaceae*

This plant is grown extensively in Hawaii and is highly prized although it has only recently become known to the rest of the world. To extract the oil the nuts are shelled, lightly roasted and then pressed to produce a light yellow oil. 'Kukui' means 'enlightenment' in Hawaii and newborn infants were traditionally anointed with kukui nut oil to protect the skin. During a trip to Hawaii I purchased some kukui nut oil and now use it regularly – it has such a beautiful, fine, soft and silky texture.

Uses:
- *beneficial for ageing skin and wrinkles*
- *nourishing for all types of skin*
- *helps eczema and psoriasis*
- *excellent for dry and dehydrated skin*
- *relieves sunburn*
- *beneficial for acne*
- *useful for scars*
- *nourishes dry hair and skin.*

Special precautions:
None.

MACADAMIA OIL

Latin name: *Macadamia integrifolia/tetraphylla*

Family name: *Proteaceae*

The macadamia tree is native to Australia and the oil that is cold pressed from the nuts is a golden colour and has a slightly nutty aroma.

Uses:
- *nourishing for all types of skin*
- *excellent for mature, ageing skin*
- *conditions dry, coloured and permed hair*
- *relieves sunburn*
- *affords protection from the sun.*

Special precautions:
None.

NEEM OIL

Latin name: *Azadirachta indica*

Family name: *Meliaceae*

Neem oil is widely used in India – early Sanskrit medical writings refer to the benefits of neem. Modern research indicates that in the future neem will be much more widely used in the treatment of many diseases. Neem oil is extracted from the seeds and has a very powerful aroma which does not appeal to everyone. You would never use it 100 per cent but a small percentage (not more than 10 per cent) added to your carrier oil is extremely beneficial for some conditions.

Uses:
▶ *excellent for relieving itching and irritation*
▶ *add a small amount to a carrier oil to treat head lice*
▶ *treats fungal, viral and bacterial infections.*

Special precautions:
Neem is considered generally safe.

ROSEHIP OIL

Latin name: *Rosa canina*

Family name: *Rosaceae*

Rosehip oil is usually obtained by solvent extraction and is a golden reddish oil with an aroma similar to castor oil.

Uses:
▶ *encourages regeneration of the skin and therefore excellent for mature skin*
▶ *heals scars and wounds*

▶ *relieves burns*
▶ *helps eczema and psoriasis.*

Special precautions:
None.

SAFFLOWER OIL

Latin name: *Carthamus tinctorius*

Family name: *Asteraceae* (or *Compositae*)

Safflower oil is extracted by cold expression of the seeds to produce a pale yellow oil with little odour very similar to sunflower oil. The safflower plant has a long history of use and interestingly safflower seeds have been discovered in Egyptian tombs.

Uses:
▶ *useful for dry skin*
▶ *beneficial for eczema and psoriasis*
▶ *helps poor circulation*
▶ *soothes inflamed joints and bruises.*

Special precautions:
None.

SUNFLOWER OIL

Latin name: *Helianthus annus*

Family name: *Asteraceae* (or *Compositae*)

Most sunflower oil, unfortunately, is obtained by solvent extraction although a small percentage is produced by cold pressing. The oil is virtually odourless with a light texture.

Uses:
▶ *moisturizes all types of skin*
▶ *helps skin disorders such as eczema*

- *reduces acne*
- *good for oily skin*
- *beneficial for bruises.*

Special precautions:
None if the unrefined oil is used.

TAMANU OIL

Latin name: *Calophyllum inophyllum*

Family name: *Clusiaceae*

Tamanu oil is obtained by cold pressing the fruit and seeds and the oil is thick and dark greyish-green to black in colour.

Uses:
- *useful for all types of skin*
- *relieves itchy skin and conditions such as eczema and psoriasis*
- *soothes inflammation*
- *helps cracked nipples and skin*
- *stimulates the immune system*
- *tamanu oil and the essential oil ravensara (discussed in Chapter 5) have proved effective treatments for shingles.*

Special precautions:
None.

TEST YOUR KNOWLEDGE

1 *Why is mineral oil, such as commercial baby oil, not suitable for aromatherapy?*

2 *Name four factors to bear in mind when choosing a carrier oil.*

3 *Choose three oils from the following list which are often used on their own:*
    a *sweet almond*
    b *apricot kernel*
    c *avocado*
    d *grapeseed*
    e *jojoba*
    f *wheatgerm*

4 *Which carrier oil is often taken in capsule form for a wide variety of conditions?*

5 *Which carrier oil contains high levels of vitamin E?*
    a *jojoba*
    b *olive*
    c *wheatgerm*

5

A–Z of essential oils

In this chapter you will learn:

- *about the physical, emotional and spiritual effects of over 50 essential oils.*

There are hundreds of essential oils that are available to the perfume and flavour industries although not all are safe for aromatherapy use. In this chapter I explore more than 50 essential oils commonly used in mainstream aromatherapy, outlining how each essential oil works upon the body and mind, as well as the spirit. I have worked extensively with essential oils treating tens of thousands of clients and have used them for all the conditions I have indicated and therefore can recommend them. If you are using aromatherapy at home and on family and friends, start off by buying just a few essential oils and gradually add more to your collection.

Insight

Unless you are a professional aromatherapist it is not necessary to buy an extensive range of essential oils all at once. Just a few essential oils are all you need to meet your everyday needs and to treat a wide range of common ailments. I suggest you start off with the essential oils listed in Only got a minute? – bergamot, cajeput, chamomile, cypress, geranium, lavender, lemon, peppermint and rosemary.

In my essential oil profiles, for simplification, I have included 'keywords' which indicate at a glance the main effects of each oil.

Any precautions which must be observed are listed at the end of each essential oil.

ANGELICA SEED

Latin name:	*Angelica archangelica*
Family:	*Umbelleferae* (or *Apiaceae*)
Method of extraction:	Steam distillation from the seeds and also from the roots and rhizomes.
Principal constituents:	Phellandrene, pinene, limonene, linalool, borneol.
Origin:	Native to Europe and Siberia. Cultivated in Belgium, Hungary, Germany, Holland, France and England.
Aroma:	Seed – clear, spicy, sweet, fresh.
	Root – earthy, herbaceous, rich, woody.
Colour:	Seed – almost colourless.
	Root – pale yellow to orange-brown.

Principal properties and indications – keywords
- Immuno-boosting
- Promotes fertility
- Stress-relieving
- Strengthening

Circulatory system
- ▶ *An excellent oil for purifying the blood and for stimulating the circulation as well as the immune system.*
- ▶ *Strengthens the heart.*
- ▶ *Reduces fever.*

Digestive system
- ▶ *Stimulates the appetite and therefore useful after illness or for conditions such as anorexia.*
- ▶ *Relieves flatulence and indigestion.*

Genito-urinary system
- ▶ *Helpful for cystitis and urinary infections.*
- ▶ *Relieves painful periods.*
- ▶ *Reduces fluid retention.*

▶ *Promotes fertility (the Chinese use angelica for infertility and female disorders).*

Muscles/joints
▶ *Beneficial for arthritis, rheumatism and gout.*

Nervous system
▶ *Excellent for extreme exhaustion and convalescence.*
▶ *Helps ME and glandular fever.*
▶ *All stress-related disorders.*
▶ *Recommended for weak, nervous individuals.*
▶ *Used for migraine headaches.*

Respiratory system
▶ *Renowned for its beneficial effects on bronchial problems.*
▶ *Use for coughs, colds and flu.*

Skin
▶ *Excellent for skin conditions.*
▶ *Beneficial for eczema and psoriasis.*
▶ *Clears congested and sluggish skin.*
▶ *Helpful for cellulite.*

Effects on spirit
▶ *Angelica seed enables you to become more in touch with and to develop your intuition. It also helps those who are fearful or weak.*

Special precautions
▶ *Angelica root oil is highly phototoxic so strong sunlight should be avoided immediately after treatment. Angelica seed oil is not phototoxic and is the preferred essential oil for aromatherapy.*

Insight

Angelica seed is particularly recommended for those who feel tired and weak after a period of prolonged stress or illness.

BASIL (FRENCH)/SWEET BASIL/COMMON BASIL

Latin name:	*Ocimum basilicum*
Family:	*Lamiaceae* (or *Labiatae*)
Method of extraction:	Steam distillation of the flowering tops of plant.
Principal constituents:	Linalool, cineole, methyl chavicol.
Origin:	Native to tropical Asia and the Middle East. Cultivated throughout Europe particularly in France, Egypt, Italy, Bulgaria, Hungary.
Aroma:	Clear, spicy, sweet, fresh.
Colour:	Colourless to pale yellow.

Principal properties and indications – keywords

- Awakening
- Clarifying
- Decongestive
- Stimulating
- Strengthening
- Uplifting

Digestive system

▶ *Recommended for digestive disorders.*

▶ *Highly beneficial for relieving difficult and painful digestion.*

▶ *Useful for flatulence, gastric spasms, nausea and vomiting.*

Genito-urinary system

▶ *Recommended for delayed menstruation, scanty periods and menstrual cramps.*

Muscles/joints

▶ *Relieves muscle spasms, cramp, gout, arthritis and rheumatism.*

▶ *Use after exercise for tired muscles.*

Nervous system

▶ *Probably one of the best nerve tonics as basil uplifts, clarifies, strengthens and restores.*

▶ *Use for mental fatigue and inability to concentrate as it is reputed to clear the head.*

▶ *Relieves nervous tension, depression and nervous exhaustion.*

Respiratory system
▶ *All respiratory problems including asthma, bronchitis, coughs, colds and whooping cough.*
▶ *Excellent for clearing the head.*
▶ *Use for catarrh, earache, nasal polyps, rhinitis, sinusitis, head colds, headaches and migraines.*

Skin
▶ *Effective as an insect repellent especially for wasps and mosquitoes.*

Effects on spirit
▶ *Uplifts and awakens the spirit, encouraging the development of intuition.*

Special precautions
▶ *Take care in pregnancy (although toxicity is unproven).*
▶ *Use in low dilution with sensitive skin (although sensitivity is rare).*
▶ *Do not use Exotic basil, also known as Comoran or Reunion basil, which has a higher percentage of methyl chavicol content making it unsuitable for use in aromatherapy. Exotic basil oil is pale yellow to pale green with a herbaceous, camphor-like, aniseed-like aroma.*

Insight
Use basil as an inhalant to clear away catarrh and sinusitis. Basil is an excellent oil for clearing the head and it aids concentration and focuses the mind. Burn it to help you study!

BENZOIN

Latin name:	*Styrax benzoin*
Family:	*Styraceae*
Method of extraction:	Solvent extraction.
Principal constituents:	Benzoic acid, vanillin, coniferyl benzoate.

Origin:	Sumatra benzoin – Java and Malaysia.
	Siam benzoin – Cambodia, China, Laos, Thailand and Vietnam.
Aroma:	Vanilla-like.
Colour:	Brownish and viscous as it is produced by solvent extraction.

Principal properties and indications – keywords

- Comforting
- Gets things moving
- Healing
- Soothing
- Warming

Circulatory system
▶ *Stimulates the circulation.*
▶ *Warms and regulates the heart.*

Genito-urinary system
▶ *Relieves all vaginal infections, discharges and irritations such as cystitis.*
▶ *Reduces fluid retention.*

Muscles/joints
▶ *Combats arthritis, gout, rheumatism and fibrositis.*

Nervous system
▶ *A warming oil that beings comfort to the recently bereaved and sad, lonely or depressed individuals.*
▶ *Instils positivity.*

Respiratory system
▶ *Benzoin is a component of Friar's Balsam and is valuable for respiratory problems such as asthma, bronchitis, colds, coughs, flu, laryngitis and throat infections.*

Skin
▶ *Excellent for cracked and chapped skin.*
▶ *Soothes redness, irritation and dermatitis and encourages healing of sores and wounds.*

Effects on spirit

▶ *Protects the spirit. Uplifting and beneficial for the heart and solar plexus.*

Special precautions

▶ *Do not take internally (it is not a distilled oil).*

Insight

Benzoin is a very useful addition to any foot or hand cream. It soothes redness and irritation and prevents and treats cracked and chapped hands and feet.

BERGAMOT

Latin name:	*Citrus bergamia*
Family:	*Rutaceae*
Method of extraction:	Cold expression of the peel.
Principal constituents:	Linalyl acetate, linalool, limonene.
Origin:	Native to tropical Asia. Cultivated in Corsica, Italy and the Ivory Coast.
Aroma:	Light, fresh, citrus.
Colour:	Green.

Principal properties and indications – keywords

- Antidepressant
- Antiseptic
- Balancing
- Uplifting

Digestive system

▶ *A tonic for the digestion stimulating a poor appetite and alleviating gas, colic and indigestion.*

▶ *Relieves halitosis (bad breath) when used as a gargle.*

▶ *Particularly useful for digestive problems linked with emotional stress.*

▶ *Recommended for eating disorders such as anorexia and bulimia.*

Genito-urinary system

▶ *Has a strong affinity for this system helping cystitis, vaginal discharges, thrush and pruritis (itching) – use in the early stages for maximum benefit.*

Nervous system
▶ *Sedative yet uplifting.*
▶ *Ideal for all states of anxiety, depression and stress-related conditions.*

Respiratory system
▶ *Relieves sore throats, tonsillitis, colds, flu and all respiratory infections.*

Skin
▶ *Improves all stress-related skin conditions such as eczema and psoriasis.*
▶ *Use for contagious conditions such as scabies, chickenpox and head lice.*
▶ *Helps oily skin, acne, spots, boils and herpes.*
▶ *Effective for cold sores, chickenpox and shingles.*

Effects on spirit
▶ *Uplifts and refreshes the spirit encouraging a joyful approach to life.*

Special precautions
▶ *Do not apply prior to sunbathing as it increases the photosensitivity of the skin due to its bergaptene content, which accelerates tanning.*

Insight
Bergamot is a very uplifting oil and is renowned for its ability to treat anxiety and all stress-related disorders. A great oil to put in your bath or burn when you're feeling low.

If, like me, you are a fan of Earl Grey tea you will recognize the aroma as the leaves of the plant are used in the manufacture of the tea.

BLACK PEPPER

Latin name:	*Piper nigrum*
Family:	*Piperaceae*
Method of extraction:	Steam distillation of the dried, crushed black peppercorns.
Principal constituents:	Mostly terpenes including caryophyllene, pinene, sabinene, limonene.
Origin:	Native to Southern India. Cultivated in India, Indonesia, Malaysia, China and Madagascar.
Aroma:	Sharp, spicy, hot, warming.
Colour:	Clear to pale, greenish-yellow.

Principal properties and indications – keywords
- Detoxifying
- Eliminative
- 'Get-up-and-go'
- Restorative
- Stimulant
- Tonic
- Warming

Circulatory system
- ▶ *A warming oil excellent for poor circulation.*
- ▶ *Recommended for anaemia and after heavy bleeding.*
- ▶ *Helpful for chilblains.*

Digestive system
- ▶ *Dispels toxins from the digestive system alleviating colic, constipation and food poisoning.*
- ▶ *Stimulates a poor appetite.*
- ▶ *Restores tone to the colon.*

Muscles/joints
- ▶ *Restores tone to the skeletal system.*
- ▶ *Relieves muscular aches and pains, neuralgia, stiffness, arthritis, rheumatism, sprains and strains.*

▶ *Recommended prior to training to improve performance and afterwards to prevent pain and stiffness.*

Nervous system
▶ *Stimulates the mind, aiding concentration and strengthening the nerves.*
▶ *Useful for coldness, indifference and apathy.*
▶ *Recommended for impotence.*

Respiratory system
▶ *Drives out coughs, colds, chills, catarrh and phlegm.*

Effects on spirit
▶ *A grounding oil which also encourages change and instils positive thoughts and actions.*
▶ *Enables us to express love and compassion.*

Special precautions
▶ *None.*

Insight
A great 'get-up-and-go' oil that strengthens the nerves, combats apathy and fills you with courage and stamina. Black pepper is one of my favourite oils for boosting the circulation.

CAJEPUT

Latin name:	*Melaleuca leucodendron/cajeputi*
Family:	*Myrtaceae*
Method of extraction:	Steam distillation of the twigs and leaves of the tree.
Principal constituents:	Cineole, limonene, pinene, terpineol.
Origin:	Native to Malaysia and Indonesia and cultivated in Indonesia, Malaysia, Philippines, Vietnam, Java and Southeast Asia.

| Aroma: | Penetrating, medicinal, camphor-like, peppery odour. |
| Colour: | Pale yellow to green. |

Principal properties and indications – keywords

- Antiseptic
- Decongestive
- Penetrating
- Stimulating
- Warming

Digestive system
▶ *Helpful for gastric spasms, upset stomachs and diarrhoea.*
▶ *Soothes inflammation of the intestines.*

Genito-urinary system
▶ *Alleviates all urinary infections such as cystitis and urethritis.*

Muscles/joints
▶ *Excellent for pain relief.*
▶ *Use for all aches, painful joints, arthritis, rheumatism, gout, sciatica, sprains and strains.*
▶ *Recommended for sports injuries.*

Nervous system
▶ *Clears and stimulates the mind and aids concentration.*
▶ *Alleviates fatigue and drowsiness.*

Respiratory system
▶ *Valuable for the respiratory system as an inhalant and a chest rub.*
▶ *Reduces high temperatures.*
▶ *Encourages the expulsion of mucus.*
▶ *Useful as a gargle for laryngitis and throat infections.*
▶ *Excellent as an inhalation for sinusitis and catarrh.*

Skin
▶ *Useful for oily skin, spots, boils and head lice.*

Effects on spirit
▶ *Elevates the spirit and encourages the creation of new pathways.*

Special precautions
- ▶ *Take care with sensitive skin (although irritation unproven).*
- ▶ *Use in a low dilution.*

> **Insight**
>
> My favourite decongestant which has a gentler action than the more commonly used eucalyptus oil. Use the inhalation method to loosen mucus and use cajeput in a chest rub for coughs and colds.

CARDAMOM

Latin name:	*Elettaria cardamomum*
Family:	*Zingiberaceae*
Method of extraction:	Steam distillation from the dried ripe fruit (seeds).
Principal constituents:	Cineole, terpinyl acetate. Also limonene, sabinene, pinene, zingiberene, linalyl acetate.
Origin:	Native to Asia and the Middle East. Mainly produced in India, Europe, Sri Lanka and Guatemala.
Aroma:	Sweet, spicy, warming.
Colour:	Colourless to pale yellow.

Principal properties and indications – keywords
- Digestive
- Stimulating
- Tonic
- Warming

Circulatory system
- ▶ *Beneficial for poor circulation.*
- ▶ *Detoxifies the lymph.*

Digestive system
- ▶ *Stimulates a poor appetite.*
- ▶ *Useful for digestive disturbances including indigestion, spasmodic pains, nausea, flatulence and constipation.*

Genito-urinary system
▶ *Helpful for fluid retention.*

Muscles/joints
▶ *Combats muscular aches and pains.*
▶ *Alleviates cramps.*
▶ *Helpful for sciatica due to its pain-relieving properties.*

Nervous system
▶ *Excellent tonic for the nerves.*
▶ *Recommended for depression.*
▶ *Combats mental fatigue.*
▶ *Helps poor concentration and memory loss.*
▶ *Alleviates mental strain.*
▶ *Instils confidence, courage and strength.*

Respiratory system
▶ *Relieves coughs and colds.*
▶ *Combats catarrhal conditions.*

Effects on spirit
▶ *Encourages you to find your sense of direction and strengthens your purpose and will.*
▶ *Instils inspiration.*

Special precautions
▶ *None.*

Insight
A warming tonic especially in the winter months. Cardamom is also an excellent choice for the digestive system. Try a compress or a gentle aromamassage of the abdomen to alleviate pain.

CARROT SEED

Latin name:	*Daucus carota*
Family:	*Umbelliferae* (or *Apiaceae*)

Method of extraction:	Steam distillation of the dried seeds.
Principal constituents:	Carotol, pinene, limonene.
Origin:	Europe.
Aroma:	Fresh, earthy, slightly spicy.
Colour:	Amber to pale orangey-brown.

Principal properties and indications – keywords

- Detoxifying
- Revitalizing
- Stimulating
- Tonic

Circulatory system

▶ *Stimulates poor circulation and purifies and detoxifies blood and lymph.*

▶ *Helpful for anaemia.*

▶ *Boosts the immune system.*

Digestive system

▶ *Alleviates constipation, irritable bowel syndrome, flatulence and liver problems.*

▶ *Aids digestion.*

▶ *Useful for eating disorders such as anorexia.*

Genito-urinary system

▶ *Combats fluid retention and cystitis.*

▶ *Regulates the menstrual cycle and balances the hormones.*

Nervous system

▶ *Recommended for confusion and indecision – it enables us to see situations more clearly.*

▶ *Stimulating and revitalizing.*

Skin

▶ *Useful for skin problems, it is a tonic increasing the elasticity of the skin.*

▶ *Ideal for mature skins.*

▶ *Reduces scarring, for instance after acne.*

▶ *Improves the complexion of the skin.*

▶ *Revitalizes tired, dull, lifeless skin.*

Effects on spirit
▶ *Strengthens inner vision.*
▶ *Spurs us on to get the most out of life.*

Special precautions
▶ *None.*

Insight

I highly recommend carrot seed for all types of skin. Add three drops to 10 ml carrier oil or 10 g cream to create a wonderful moisturiser to prevent and reduce wrinkling. One of my favourite recipes for a facial oil includes carrot seed, frankincense and neroli.

CEDARWOOD, ATLAS

Latin name:	*Cedrus atlantica*
Family:	*Pinaceae*
Method of extraction:	Steam distillation of the wood, stumps and sawdust.
Principal constituents:	Cedrene, atlantone, atlantol, himachalene.
Origin:	Native to the Atlas Mountains of Algeria and Morocco. Cultivated mainly in Morocco.
Aroma:	Warm, woody, heady, sweet.
Colour:	Orangey-yellow to deep amber.

Principal properties and indications – keywords
- Calming
- Detoxifying
- Peaceful
- Soothing
- Warming

Circulatory system
▶ *Excellent for poor circulation.*
▶ *Recommended for blocked-up arteries (arteriosclerosis) and stimulates the breakdown of accumulated fats.*
▶ *Decongests the lymphatic system.*

Genito-urinary system

▶ *Eases vaginal discharges and infections.*
▶ *Recommended for fluid retention, burning pains and itching.*

Nervous system

▶ *Beneficial for all states of nervous tension, instilling peace and tranquillity.*
▶ *Good for clogged-up individuals.*
▶ *A useful aid for meditation.*
▶ *Combats lethargy and nervous debility.*
▶ *Instils confidence.*
▶ *Enables us to cope with life's stresses and strains.*

Respiratory system

▶ *Excellent for breaking up catarrh and expelling mucus.*

Skin

▶ *Helpful for cellulite, oily skin, acne and chronic conditions.*
▶ *Balances the production of sebum.*
▶ *Reputed to strengthen hair growth.*

Effects on spirit

▶ *Enhances spirituality and has a stabilizing effect on our energies when they are thrown out of balance.*
▶ *Gives us immovable strength.*

Special precautions

▶ *Avoid when pregnant.*
▶ *Do not use on babies and young children.*

Insight

Cedarwood brings peace, harmony and tranquillity. Use it in the bath or in a burner when you feel stressed and also as an aid to meditation.

CHAMOMILE, GERMAN/BLUE

Latin name:	*Matricaria Chamomilla/recutita*
Family:	*Asteraceae (or Compositae)*
Method of extraction:	Steam distillation of the flower heads.
Principal constituents:	Chamazulene, bisabolol oxide.
Origin:	German/blue chamomile is native to Europe and is cultivated in Hungary and Eastern Europe. Hungary is the main producer.
Aroma:	Intense, pungent aroma (some people prefer the sweeter aroma of Roman chamomile).
Colour:	Deep inky-blue which easily distinguishes it from Roman chamomile.

Principal properties and indications – keywords
- Antiallergenic
- Anti-inflammatory
- Balancing
- Calming
- Children
- Sedative

Circulatory system
▶ *Excellent for stimulating the white blood cells and thus boosting the immune system.*
▶ *Reduces fever.*

Digestive system
▶ *Valuable for children's problems such as colic and diarrhoea.*
▶ *Recommended for poor appetite, slow painful digestion, indigestion and ulcers.*
▶ *Combats nausea.*
▶ *Stimulates the liver and gall bladder.*

Genito-urinary system
▶ *Beneficial for urinary infections such as cystitis.*
▶ *Balances the menstrual cycle.*

- ▶ *Relieves painful menstruation.*
- ▶ *Recommended for PMS and the menopause.*

Muscular/joints
- ▶ *Useful for all aches and pains.*
- ▶ *Excellent for inflamed joints.*
- ▶ *Beneficial for sprains and strains and inflamed tendons.*
- ▶ *Relieves headaches and migraine.*

Nervous system
- ▶ *Relaxes the nerves.*
- ▶ *Excellent for anxiety and stress.*
- ▶ *Combats insomnia.*
- ▶ *Releases anger and frustration.*
- ▶ *Provides comfort and support while grieving.*

Skin
- ▶ *A 'must-have' for skin that is inflamed or prone to allergies. It reduces histamine-induced tissue reactions.*
- ▶ *Valuable for eczema and psoriasis.*
- ▶ *Soothes burns and acne.*
- ▶ *Beneficial for sensitive skin.*
- ▶ *Reduces the redness of the skin.*

Effects on spirit
- ▶ *Heals the aura and counteracts a troubled soul.*

Special precautions
- ▶ *None. Suitable for even babies and young children.*

Insight

An invaluable oil for calming the mind, easing anxiety and irritability. I highly recommend blue chamomile for the menopause and for all skin problems, especially allergies.

CHAMOMILE, ROMAN

Latin name:	*Anthemis nobilis/Chamaemelum nobile*
Family:	*Asteraceae (or Compositae)*

Method of extraction:	Steam distillation from the flowering tops.
Principal constituents:	75–80 per cent esters including angelates. Also chamazulene, cineole, pinene and caryophyllene.
Origin:	Native to Southern and Western Europe and is cultivated in England, Belgium, France and Hungary.
Aroma:	Warm, sweet, fresh, apple-like.
Colour:	Pale blue.

Principal properties and indications – keywords

- Anti-inflammatory
- Calming
- Children
- Sedative

Circulatory system

▶ *Useful for boosting the immune system and reducing susceptibility to infection.*

▶ *Indicated for anaemia.*

Digestive system

▶ *Calms the digestive system easing gas and colic.*

▶ *Relieves indigestion and diarrhoea.*

▶ *Excellent for children's digestive problems.*

▶ *Eases inflammation in the bowels and thus important for IBS (irritable bowel syndrome).*

▶ *Boosts a poor appetite.*

▶ *Useful for the liver and gall bladder.*

Genito-urinary system

▶ *Ideal for the menopause and PMS.*

▶ *Balances the menstrual cycle.*

▶ *Helpful for painful and scanty menstruation.*

▶ *Excellent for nervous menstrual problems.*

Muscular/joints

▶ *Useful for inflamed joints and tendons.*

▶ *Relieves pain.*

▶ *Beneficial for gout.*

- *Combats headaches, migraine and neuralgia.*
- *Relaxes muscles, especially when associated with nervous tension.*

Nervous system
- *Exerts a pronounced calming effect on the nervous system and mind.*
- *Ideal for oversensitive individuals and those prone to hysteria.*
- *Soothes restlessness, irritability and impatience.*
- *Alleviates anxiety and stress.*
- *Useful for insomnia.*

Respiratory system
- *Recommended for nervous asthma due to its calming effect.*

Skin
- *Beneficial for all types of skin including sensitive, red and dry skin.*
- *Suitable for eczema and psoriasis.*
- *Soothes irritated and inflamed skin.*
- *Useful for cracked nipples.*
- *Recommended after shaving.*

Effects on spirit
- *Promotes a harmonious, peaceful and joyful spirit.*

Special precautions
- *None. A safe oil, suitable for babies, young children and highly sensitive individuals.*

Insight
A must-have oil for babies and children. Chamomile eases colic, soothes restlessness and temper tantrums and promotes a good night's sleep.

CINNAMON

Latin name:	*Cinnamomum zeylanicum/verum*
Family:	*Lauraceae*
Method of extraction:	Steam distillation from the leaves (cinnamon leaf) and from the bark.
Principal constituents:	Cinnamon *leaf* – eugenol, eugenol acetate, cinnamaldehyde, benzyl benzoate.
	Cinnamon *bark* – cinnamic aldehyde, eugenol, benzyl benzoate, pinene, cineole, linalool.
	(*Do not use cinnamon bark.*)
Origin:	Native to Sri Lanka, India and Madagascar. Also cultivated in Jamaica and Africa.
Aroma:	Cinnamon *leaf* – hot and spicy and warming.
	Cinnamon *bark* – strong, warm, spicy aroma.
Colour:	Cinnamon *leaf* – yellow to brownish-yellow.
	Cinnamon *bark* – light amber.

Principal properties and indications – keywords

- Digestive
- Stimulating
- Tonic
- Warming

Circulatory system

▶ *Stimulates the circulation.*

▶ *Improves a poor immune system.*

Digestive system

▶ *Encourages a sluggish digestion.*

▶ *Stimulates the appetite.*

▶ *Relieves indigestion, nausea and flatulence and warms the stomach.*

▶ *Helps combat diarrhoea, spasms and constipation.*

▶ *Recommended for candida.*

Genito-urinary system

▶ *Useful for vaginal discharges.*

▶ *Beneficial for scanty menstruation.*

▶ *Stimulates contractions in childbirth.*

Muscles/joints
▶ *Alleviates aches and pains and rheumatism.*

Nervous system
▶ *Combats mental fatigue.*
▶ *Useful for stress-related conditions and nervous exhaustion.*

Respiratory system
▶ *Beneficial for coughs, colds, flu and chills.*

Effects on spirit
▶ *Uplifts the spirit.*

Special precautions
▶ *Cinnamon bark is highly irritating to the skin and mucous membranes and therefore cinnamon leaf is the preferred essential oil for aromatherapy. Use cinnamon leaf with care in a low concentration.*
▶ *Avoid in pregnancy.*
▶ *Do not use on young children.*

Insight
One of my favourite oils to burn at Christmas, cinnamon creates a warm and joyful atmosphere.

CITRONELLA

Latin name:	*Cymbopogon nardus*
Family:	*Poaceae* (or *Gramineae*)
Method of extraction:	Steam distillation from the grass (dried, part-dried or fresh).
Principal constituents:	Geraniol, citronellol, citronellal, limonene, camphene.
Origin:	Cultivated in Sri Lanka.
Aroma:	Fresh, strong, grassy, lemony aroma.
Colour:	Yellow to brownish-yellow.

Principal properties and indications – keywords
- Clearing
- Insect repellent
- Refreshing
- Stimulating

Digestive system
- ▶ *Helpful for poor and sluggish digestion.*
- ▶ *Stimulates the appetite.*
- ▶ *Combats candida.*

Genito-urinary system
- ▶ *Useful for fluid retention.*

Muscles/joints
- ▶ *Relieves muscular aches and pains.*

Nervous system
- ▶ *Banishes extreme fatigue, lethargy and exhaustion.*
- ▶ *Clears the mind.*

Respiratory system
- ▶ *Helpful for colds and flu.*

Skin
- ▶ *Refreshes sweaty and tired feet.*
- ▶ *Combats excessive perspiration and oily skin.*
- ▶ *Extensively used as an insect repellent.*

Effects on spirit
- ▶ *Uplifts the spirit.*

Special precautions
- ▶ *Avoid using on sensitive skin as it may cause sensitization.*

Insight

Citronella is well known for its ability to deter insects. It is often used in burners and sprays. A good oil to pack in your suitcase! You can also put a drop on cotton wool and place in your drawers to deter moths.

CLARY SAGE

Latin name:	*Salvia sclarea*
Family:	*Lamiaceae (or Labiatae)*
Method of extraction:	Steam distillation of the flowering tops and leaves.
Principal constituents:	Linalyl acetate, linalool.
Origin:	Nature to the Mediterranean and cultivated in Europe especially Russia, Britain and Morocco.
Aroma:	Sweet, heady, floral.
Colour:	Colourless to pale yellow.

Principal properties and indications – keywords
- Euphoric
- Intoxicating
- Relaxing
- Tonic

Circulatory system
▶ *Excellent for reducing the blood pressure and counteracting palpitations.*

Genito-urinary system
▶ *Recommended for childbirth since it encourages labour yet promotes relaxation.*
▶ *Tonic for the womb.*
▶ *Balances the hormones, reducing PMS.*
▶ *Relieves the pain of menstrual cramps.*
▶ *Beneficial for the menopause.*

Nervous system
▶ *Exerts a euphoric–sedative effect and indicated for overactive and panicky states of mind.*
▶ *Induces a sense of well-being and optimism and creates a padding between you and the outside world.*
▶ *Suitable for all stress-related disorders and general debility whether physical, mental, nervous or sexual.*
▶ *Of assistance for those endeavouring to withdraw from drugs.*

Skin

▶ *Useful for soothing and cooling inflamed skin.*

▶ *Helps to balance oily skin, dandruff and stimulates hair growth.*

▶ *Prevents wrinkles from occurring.*

Effects on spirit

▶ *Valuable for instilling inner tranquillity; it uplifts the spirit.*

Special precautions

▶ *Large doses should not be taken together with alcohol which may induce a narcotic effect.*

▶ *Some say avoid during pregnancy, although there is no research to support or reject this.*

Insight

Clary sage is the ultimate euphoric. If your mind is overactive then clary sage will banish unwanted thoughts and induce a sense of calm.

CORIANDER

Latin name:	*Coriandrum sativum*
Family:	*Apiaceae* (or *Umbelliferae*)
Method of extraction:	Steam distillation from the crushed seeds.
Principal constituents:	Linalool, terpinene.
Origin:	Native to Europe and Western Asia. Most of the oil is now produced in Russia, Poland, Hungary, Holland, France and England.
Aroma:	Sweet, spicy, woody and peppery.
Colour:	Colourless or pale yellow.

Principal properties and indications – keywords

- Stimulating
- Tonic
- Warming
- Uplifting

Circulatory system
- ▶ *Excellent for poor circulation.*
- ▶ *Purifies the system of toxins.*

Digestive system
- ▶ *Stimulates the appetite and recommended for anorexia nervosa.*
- ▶ *Useful as a gargle for halitosis (bad breath).*
- ▶ *Relieves abdominal spasms, indigestion, flatulence, nausea, constipation and diarrhoea as well as other digestive upsets.*

Genito-urinary system
- ▶ *Helpful as a tonic for the uterus.*
- ▶ *Regulates the menstrual cycle.*

Muscles/joints
- ▶ *Beneficial for arthritis, gout and rheumatism.*
- ▶ *Relieves muscular aches and pains and stiffness in the joints.*

Nervous system
- ▶ *Good for nervous debility and fatigue.*
- ▶ *Improves concentration.*
- ▶ *Beneficial for sadness, loneliness and depression.*
- ▶ *Encourages optimism, creativity and confidence.*
- ▶ *Helpful for neuralgia.*

Respiratory system
- ▶ *Combats viruses, coughs, colds and flu.*

Effects on spirit
- ▶ *Uplifts the spirit.*

Special precautions
- ▶ *None.*

Insight
Use coriander in the bath on a physical level to boost the circulation and on an emotional level to dispel mental fatigue and lethargy.

CYPRESS

Latin name:	*Cupressus sempervirens*
Family:	*Cupressaceae*
Method of extraction:	Steam distillation of the needles and twigs.
Principal constituents:	Pinene, carene, terpinolene, camphene.
Origin:	Native to the Eastern Mediterranean area. Most of the oil is distilled in Spain, France and Morocco.
Aroma:	Woody, balsamic, refreshing; reminiscent of pine needles.
Colour:	Pale yellow.

Principal properties and indications – keywords
- Astringent
- Fluid-reducing
- Warming
- Tonic

Circulatory system
▶ *Renowned for reducing varicose veins and haemorrhoids.*
▶ *Exerts a restorative effect on the veins.*

Genito-urinary system
▶ *Helpful for fluid retention.*
▶ *Recommended for PMS and the menopause (ideal for hot flushes).*
▶ *Regulates the menstrual cycle.*

Nervous system
▶ *A comforting oil indicated for bereavement.*
▶ *Relieves anger, irritability and all stress-related conditions.*
▶ *Restores calm, balance and serenity.*

Respiratory system
▶ *Indicated for spasmodic coughing such as whooping cough.*
▶ *Useful for asthma and bronchitis.*

Skin
▶ *Excellent for oily skin and for reducing excessive perspiration.*
▶ *Combats cellulite.*

Effects on spirit
▶ *Helpful for coping with change and for finding your soul pathway.*

Special precautions
▶ *None.*

Insight
Cypress is the oil of change – use it when moving house, changing jobs, cutting old ties or for bereavement. Blend two drops cypress and one drop lemon in 10 ml carrier oil to prevent and alleviate varicose veins.

EUCALYPTUS

Latin name:	*Eucalyptus globulus*
Family:	*Myrtaceae*
Method of extraction:	Steam distillation of the leaves and twigs.
Principal constituents:	Cineole, pinene, cymene.
Origin:	Native to Australia and Tasmania and also cultivated in Portugal, Spain and China.
Aroma:	Fresh, camphor-like, penetrating.
Colour:	Colourless.

Principal properties and indications – keywords
- Antiseptic
- Expectorant
- Pain-relieving
- Stimulating

Circulatory system
▶ *Useful for poor circulation.*

Genito-urinary system
- *Excellent for all urinary infections, cystitis, thrush.*
- *Reduces fluid retention.*

Muscular/joints
- *Excellent for all aches and pains, arthritis and rheumatism due to its pain-relieving properties.*

Nervous system
- *Combats mental exhaustion and aids concentration.*
- *Encourages positivity.*

Respiratory system
- *Very useful as an inhalant and chest rub for all respiratory disorders.*
- *Decongests the head and chest and helps to expel mucus.*
- *Enhances breathing function.*
- *Useful for asthma, bronchitis, coughs, colds, flu, sinusitis and throat infections.*
- *Reduces fever, prevents the spread of infection and boosts the immune system.*

Skin
- *Useful for infectious skin diseases such as chickenpox and measles.*
- *Recommended for herpes, cuts and burns.*
- *Excellent insect repellent.*

Effects on spirit
- *Revives the spirit and clears past traumas.*

Special precautions
- *A powerful oil not to be massaged into babies and very young children.*
- *Store away from homoeopathic medicines.*

Insight
An invaluable oil for coughs and colds. Burn eucalyptus in your home to prevent the spread of infection.

FENNEL (SWEET)

Latin name:	*Foeniculum vulgare*
Family:	*Umbelliferae* (or *Apiaceae*)
Method of extraction:	Steam distillation of the crushed seeds.
Principal constituents:	Trans-anethole, methyl chavicol, fenchone.
Origin:	Native to the Mediterranean and cultivated mainly in Bulgaria, Germany, France, Italy and Greece.
Aroma:	Aniseed-like, strong, sweet, spicy.
Colour:	Colourless to pale yellow.

Principal properties and indications – keywords
- Detoxifying
- Digestive
- Eliminative
- Energizing
- Fluid-reducing
- Warming

Circulatory system
▶ *Excellent as a lymphatic decongestant.*

Digestive system
▶ *Marvellous for cleansing the digestive system (and all other systems too).*
▶ *Relieves constipation, flatulence and nausea.*
▶ *A helpful aid for slimming, curbing the appetite yet increasing energy levels.*

Genito-urinary system
▶ *Excellent for nursing mothers as it increases the flow of breast milk.*
▶ *Highly effective for the menopause since it encourages the body to produce its own oestrogen.*
▶ *Regulates the menstrual cycle.*
▶ *Eases fluid retention.*
▶ *Useful for urinary tract infections.*

Nervous system
▸ *Encourages the ability to see a situation clearly.*
▸ *Induces courage, strength and hope in the face of seemingly impossible hurdles.*
▸ *Recommended for addictions.*

Respiratory system
▸ *Useful for bronchitis, flu and shortness of breath.*

Skin
▸ *Indicated for toxic, dull, congested skin.*
▸ *Recommended for cellulite.*

Effects on spirit
▸ *Helpful for protection against psychic attack.*

Special precautions
▸ *Do not use bitter fennel.*
▸ *Do not use excessively on young children or epileptics.*
▸ *Avoid during pregnancy.*

Insight
Fennel is a valuable asset when dieting as it helps to curb the appetite yet increases your energy levels. It is really detoxifying too.

FRANKINCENSE

Latin name:	*Boswellia carteri*
Family:	*Burseraceae*
Method of extraction:	Steam distillation of oleo gum resin of trees obtained as teardrops.
Principal constituents:	Pinene, limonene, octyl acetate.
Origin:	Native to Northeast Africa and the Red Sea region and cultivated mainly in Somalia and Ethiopia.

Aroma:	Woody, spicy, balsamic, warming.
Colour:	Colourless to pale yellow.

Principal properties and indications – keywords

- Comforting
- Decongestive
- Expectorant
- Elevating
- Healing
- Rejuvenating

Genito-urinary system

▶ *Combats cystitis.*

▶ *Useful for all vaginal discharges.*

▶ *Beneficial during the menopause.*

Nervous system

▶ *Elevating yet soothing effect on the emotions.*

▶ *Allows past traumas and anxieties to fade away.*

▶ *Instils peace and calm and is an excellent aid for meditation.*

▶ *Useful for those who fear change.*

▶ *Alleviates stress-related conditions.*

Respiratory system

▶ *Ideal for asthma and other respiratory disorders. It has both physical and emotional benefits.*

▶ *Encourages the breathing to slow down and deepen.*

Skin

▶ *Excellent remedy for all types of skin.*

▶ *Rejuvenates and revitalizes mature skin and wrinkles and helps to prevent ageing.*

▶ *Reduces scars and stretch marks.*

Effects on spirit

▶ *Valuable for achieving heightened states of spiritual awareness and bringing one closer to the Divine.*

Special precautions
▶ *None.*

....

Insight

An excellent aid for meditation as it induces a heightened spiritual awareness. Frankincense also allows us to release, let go of the past and move on.

....

GERANIUM

Latin name:	*Pelargonium graveolens*
Family:	*Geraniaceae*
Method of extraction:	Steam distillation of the leaves, stalks and flowers.
Principal constituents:	Citronellol, geraniol, linalool, citronellyl formate, geranyl formate.
Origin:	Native to South Africa but cultivated mainly in Reunion (Bourbon) and Egypt.
Aroma:	Sweet, rosy, leafy.
Colour:	Greenish.

Principal properties and indications – keywords
- Antidepressant
- Balancing
- Fluid-reducing
- Healing
- Uplifting

Circulatory system
▶ *Helpful for varicose veins and haemorrhoids.*
▶ *Effective for stopping bleeding.*
▶ *Stimulates the lymphatic system.*

Genito-urinary system
▶ *Excellent for the menopause and PMS.*
▶ *Balances the hormones and combats hot flushes.*
▶ *Reduces fluid retention.*
▶ *Recommended for tension and depression.*
▶ *Helpful for cystitis.*

Nervous system

- ▶ *Wonderfully balancing for the nerves.*
- ▶ *Dispels anxiety, depression and nervous tension.*
- ▶ *Helps infertility problems.*

Skin

- ▶ *Very balancing for all types of skin – inflamed, oily, dry, combination and mature.*
- ▶ *Recommended for eczema, dermatitis, burns, infectious skin diseases and cellulite.*
- ▶ *Excellent for head lice and as an insect repellent.*

Effects on spirit

- ▶ *Valuable for uplifting the spirit.*

Special precautions

- ▶ *None.*

Insight

Geranium is one of my favourite oils to balance the hormones. A must-have for PMT and the menopause. Put a few drops on a tissue, take a few deep breaths and put it in your pocket so that you can continue to inhale the aroma throughout the day.

GINGER

Latin name:	*Zingiber officinale*
Family:	*Zingerberaceae*
Method of extraction:	Steam distillation of the dried ground rhizomes.
Principal constituents:	Zingiberene, sesquiphellandrene, ar-curcumene.
Origin:	Native to Southern Asia and cultivated in India, China, Australia, Southeast Asia and Africa.
Aroma:	Aromatic, hot, spicy.
Colour:	Pale yellow to light amber.

Principal properties and indications – keywords

- Digestive
- Fiery
- Pain-relieving
- Stimulant
- Warming

Circulatory system

▶ *Highly effective for stimulating poor circulation.*

▶ *Recommended for varicose veins and high cholesterol.*

Digestive system

▶ *Excellent for all digestive problems especially nausea (travel, chemotherapy, early morning sickness).*

▶ *Useful for diarrhoea, constipation, hangover, indigestion, flatulence, abdominal distension, loss of appetite and stomach cramps.*

Muscles/joints

▶ *Indicated for all muscular aches and pains.*

▶ *Alleviates arthritis, cramps, rheumatism, sprains and strains. Ginger works particularly well when these conditions are aggravated by damp.*

Nervous system

▶ *A warming, uplifting oil for counteracting coldness and indifference, apathy, lethargy and nervous exhaustion.*

▶ *Useful for weak-minded individuals.*

▶ *Aids concentration and memory and boosts confidence.*

Respiratory system

▶ *Excellent for coughs and colds.*

▶ *Recommended for catarrh, bronchitis, sinusitis and sore throats.*

Effects on spirit

▶ *A grounding oil which brings balance and increases our inner strength and will.*

Special precautions

▶ *Use in low dilutions if the skin is hypersensitive. At normal dosage no irritation will occur.*

Ginger is well known for its warming effects and treatment of digestive problems. Use a couple of drops on a tissue or handkerchief to combat travel sickness.

GRAPEFRUIT

Latin name:	*Citrus paradisi*
Family:	*Rutaceae*
Method of extraction:	Cold expression of the peel of the fruit.
Principal constituent:	Limonene.
Origin:	Native to tropical Asia and cultivated in the USA, Israel, Brazil and Nigeria.
Aroma:	Fresh, sweet, refreshing.
Colour:	Yellow to greenish-yellow.

Principal properties and indications – keywords
- Antidepressant
- Detoxifying
- Refreshing
- Uplifting

Circulatory system
▶ *Excellent for purifying the blood.*
▶ *Useful for unclogging the lymphatic system.*

Digestive system
▶ *An excellent aid to digestion and for detox diets.*
▶ *Useful for obesity, liver and gall bladder problems.*
▶ *Recommended for those who comfort eat.*

Muscles/joints
▶ *Valuable for arthritis, gout, rheumatism.*
▶ *Useful before and after exercise for preventing stiffness in the muscles and joints.*

Nervous system
▶ *Uplifts the mind, helping to lift depression and inducing euphoria.*
▶ *Helpful for dispelling bitterness and resentment.*

▶ *Beneficial for nervous exhaustion and stress relief.*
▶ *Increases self-esteem.*

Respiratory system
▶ *Alleviates coughs, colds, flu and glandular fever.*

Skin
▶ *Useful for oily and congested skin, acne and cellulite.*
▶ *Exerts a tonic effect on the scalp.*

Effects on spirit
▶ *Uplifts the spirit.*

Special precautions
▶ *None.*

Insight
Use grapefruit to cleanse and tone. I highly recommend using
it in the bath when detoxing and I recommend one drop
grapefruit, one drop fennel and one drop juniper in 10 ml
carrier oil to reduce cellulite.

HYSSOP

Latin name:	*Hyssopus officinalis*
Family:	*Lamiaceae* (or *Labiatae*)
Method of extraction:	Steam distillation from the leaves and flowering tops.
Principal constituents:	Pinocamphone, isopinocamphone, pinene.
Origin:	Native to the Mediterranean area. Cultivated mainly in Hungary and France and also in Albania and the former Yugoslavia.
Aroma:	Warm, sweet, herbaceous, slightly spicy penetrating aroma.
Colour:	Pale yellow to greenish-yellow.

Principal properties and indications – keywords

- Cleansing
- Digestive
- Purifying
- Regulating
- Stimulating

Circulatory system
- ▶ *Regulates the blood pressure.*
- ▶ *Helpful for improving poor circulation.*

Digestive system
- ▶ *A useful tonic for the digestive system.*
- ▶ *Alleviates bloating, constipation and flatulence.*
- ▶ *Stimulates the appetite, combats indigestion and improves the digestion generally.*

Genito-urinary system
- ▶ *Beneficial for scanty or absent menstruation.*
- ▶ *Relieves fluid retention.*

Muscles/joints
- ▶ *Beneficial for arthritis, rheumatism and gout.*
- ▶ *Reduces swellings and bruises.*

Nervous system
- ▶ *Combats anxiety and stress, exhaustion and fatigue.*
- ▶ *Useful for clearing the head and improving poor concentration and memory.*

Respiratory system
- ▶ *Excellent for all chest problems such as bronchitis, asthma and coughs.*
- ▶ *Helpful for sinusitis and hayfever.*
- ▶ *Good for sore throats and tonsillitis.*

Skin
- ▶ *Helps to disperse toxins.*
- ▶ *Useful for oily, congested skin and acne.*
- ▶ *Alleviates eczema and dermatitis.*

Effects on spirit

▶ *Cleanses and protects the spirit.*

Special precautions

▶ *Avoid in cases of epilepsy.*
▶ *Avoid during pregnancy.*
▶ *Do not use on babies and young children.*

....

Insight

Use hyssop for purification. It cleanses the body, clears the head and focuses the mind. Burn hyssop if you are having difficulty concentrating.

....

JASMINE

Latin name:	*Jasminum officinale*
Family:	*Oleaceae*
Method of extraction:	Solvent extraction of the flowers.
Principal constituents:	Benzyl acetate, benzyl benzoate, cis-jasmone, linalool, phytols.
Origin:	Native to China, Northern India and the Middle East. Cultivated mainly in Egypt and France.
Aroma:	Exotic, floral, heady, sensual, rich, warm.
Colour:	Orangey-brown.

Principal properties and indications – keywords

- Antidepressant
- Aphrodisiac
- Euphoric
- Healing
- Uplifting

Genito-urinary system

▶ *Highly recommended for childbirth as it helps to relieve pain, promote the birth and expel the placenta.*
▶ *Useful after childbirth since it stimulates milk production and prevents postnatal depression.*
▶ *A renowned aphrodisiac, jasmine can alleviate frigidity, impotence and premature ejaculation.*

- *Increases the sperm count.*
- *Excellent for painful menstruation, PMS and the menopause.*

Nervous system
- *A wonderful oil for problems of the nervous system, releasing anxiety, lifting sadness and depression and inducing optimism, confidence and euphoria.*
- *Counteracts apathy and indifference.*

Skin
- *Excellent for all types of skin, jasmine increases the elasticity of the skin and reduces stretch marks and scars.*
- *Beneficial for dry and sensitive skin.*

Effects on spirit
- *Liberates the spirit.*

Special precautions
- *Do not take internally (it is an absolute).*

Insight

I use jasmine extensively for nervous problems as it lifts even the darkest mood. Jasmine makes one feel optimistic and confident. Jasmine also releases inhibitions and is a powerful aphrodisiac!

JUNIPER BERRY

Latin name:	*Juniperus communis*
Family:	*Cupressaceae*
Method of extraction:	Steam distillation of crushed dried berries.
Principal constituents:	Pinene, limonene, sabinene, myrcene, cymene, terpinene, terpinen-4-ol.
Origin:	Cultivated mainly in Eastern Europe, France, Italy, Austria and Germany.
Aroma:	Fresh, woody, pine-needle like.
Colour:	Virtually colourless to very pale yellow.

Principal properties and indications – keywords

- Antiseptic
- Cleansing
- Detoxifying
- Fluid-reducing
- Purifying
- Tonic

Circulatory system

- ▶ *Renowned as a wonderful detoxifier.*
- ▶ *Beneficial for arteriosclerosis.*
- ▶ *Decongests the lymphatic system.*
- ▶ *Boosts the circulation.*

Digestive system

- ▶ *Stimulates the elimination of toxins and therefore useful for obesity, constipation and stomach upsets after too much rich food and alcohol.*

Genito-urinary system

- ▶ *Excellent for relieving fluid retention.*
- ▶ *One of the best oils for urinary infections such as cystitis.*
- ▶ *Useful for prostate problems and kidney stones.*
- ▶ *A remedy for scanty, irregular and painful menstruation.*

Muscles/joints

- ▶ *Alleviates arthritis, gout and rheumatic disorders, stimulating the elimination of uric acid and other toxins and relieving pain and stiffness.*

Nervous system

- ▶ *Ideal for emotional depletion.*
- ▶ *Clears waste from the mind just as it does from the body.*

Skin

- ▶ *Recommended for all skin conditions due to an accumulation of toxins.*
- ▶ *Invaluable for cellulite, acne, blocked pores and oily skin.*
- ▶ *Helpful for dermatitis, eczema and psoriasis.*
- ▶ *Since juniper encourages elimination, skin conditions may worsen before an improvement is seen.*

Effects on spirit
▶ *A classic remedy for purifying and cleansing the spirit and for those who are unable to move on.*
▶ *Juniper helps to clear away the residues of unwanted past traumas.*

Special precautions
▶ *Avoid during pregnancy.*
▶ *Do not use excessively where there is inflammation of the kidneys.*

Insight
Juniper clears toxins from the body, mind and spirit. Use in the bath after over-indulging and whenever you feel emotionally depleted.

LAVENDER

Latin name:	*Lavandula angustifolia/officinalis/vera*
Family:	*Lamiaceae* (or *Labiatae*)
Method of extraction:	Steam distillation of the flowering tops.
Principal constituents:	Linalyl acetate, linalool, lavandulyl acetate.
Origin:	Native to the Mediterranean area and cultivated mainly in Bulgaria and France.
Aroma:	Sweet, floral, herbaceous.
Colour:	Colourless to pale yellow.

Principal properties and indications – keywords
- Antidepressant
- Antiseptic
- Balancing
- Calming
- Healing

Circulatory system
▶ *Excellent for high blood pressure, palpitations and all other cardiac disorders exacerbated by stress.*

Digestive system

- *Good for all digestive disorders, especially in children, such as colic and diarrhoea.*
- *Useful for difficult and painful digestion, flatulence, indigestion, nausea and vomiting.*

Genito-urinary system

- *Helpful for cystitis, discharges and fluid retention.*
- *During childbirth lavender speeds up the delivery, calms the mother and purifies the air.*
- *Relieves PMS, menstrual pain and the menopause.*

Muscles/joints

- *Reduces muscular aches and pains since lavender provides pain relief, relieves spasm and reduces inflammation.*
- *Recommended for arthritis, rheumatism, cramps, sprains and strains.*

Nervous system

- *Harmonizes the nervous system.*
- *Relieves emotional stress and anxiety.*
- *Combats depression.*
- *Excellent remedy for migraines, headaches and insomnia.*

Respiratory system

- *As an immuno-booster lavender is recommended for protection against all infections.*
- *Useful for viruses, colds, coughs, flu, bronchitis, asthma and throat infections.*

Skin

- *Useful for all skin care due to its powers of rejuvenation, antiseptic, antifungal, pain-relieving, healing and balancing properties.*
- *Helps to heal bruises, burns, sunburn, acne, boils, eczema, fungal infections (e.g. athlete's foot) and psoriasis.*
- *Useful for infectious skin conditions such as scabies and chickenpox.*

- ▶ *Heals wounds and sores.*
- ▶ *Treats insect bites (apply neat).*

Effects on spirit
- ▶ *Calms and soothes an angry spirit.*
- ▶ *Helps to centre those on the wrong spiritual pathway.*

Special precautions
- ▶ *None. Lavender is used extensively on babies and children.*

Insight

Lavender is the most versatile of all essential oils and is a must-have for your first aid kit. Use it neat on cuts, burns and insect bites. Sprinkle a few drops on your pillow to combat insomnia.

LEMON

Latin name:	*Citrus limonum*
Family:	*Rutaceae*
Method of extraction:	Cold expression of the peel of the fruit.
Principal constituents:	Limonene, pinene, terpinene.
Origin:	Native to Asia and cultivated in Southern Europe, California and Florida.
Aroma:	Clean, crisp, fruity, refreshing, light.
Colour:	Pale yellow to greenish-yellow.

Principal properties and indications – keywords
- Alkaline
- Antiseptic
- Detoxifying
- Fluid-reducing
- Purifying
- Tonic

Circulatory system
- ▶ *Excellent tonic for the circulation.*
- ▶ *Stimulates and cleanses the circulatory system.*
- ▶ *Boosts the immune system accelerating recovery time.*
- ▶ *Useful for high blood pressure and arteriosclerosis.*
- ▶ *Helpful for stopping bleeding, varicose veins and haemorrhoids.*

Digestive system
- *Highly effective for the digestion as it relieves hyperacidity, stomach ulcers and liver and gall bladder congestion.*
- *Ideal for obesity and detoxification.*

Genito-urinary system
- *An excellent diuretic relieving fluid retention.*
- *Combats kidney and bladder infections and thrush.*

Muscles/joints
- *Useful for arthritis, gout and rheumatism.*

Nervous system
- *Stimulates a tired and exhausted mind, encouraging clear thinking and aiding concentration.*
- *Aids in decision making.*
- *Restores confidence.*

Respiratory system
- *Relieves asthma, bronchitis, catarrh, colds, flu, laryngitis, throat infections and sinusitis.*

Skin
- *Effective for cleaning out cuts and wounds.*
- *Reduces broken capillaries.*
- *Useful for teenage problem skin.*
- *Recommended for cellulite.*
- *Beneficial for ageing skin, brown patches, greasy skin, boils, herpes and scabies.*
- *May be applied neat to warts and verrucae.*

Effects on spirit
- *Restores strength, vitality and positivity to a depleted spirit.*
- *Spiritually cleansing.*

Special precautions
- *Avoid strong sunlight immediately after treatment.*

> ## Insight
>
> To treat warts and verrucae simply dab one drop of lemon
> on to the affected area with a cotton wool bud or pad several
> times a day.

LEMONGRASS (WEST INDIAN)

Latin name:	*Cymbopogon citratus*
Family:	*Gramineae* (or *Poaceae*)
Method of extraction:	Steam distillation of fresh, partially dried leaves.
Principal constituents:	Citral, geranial, geraniol, neral, nerol.
Origin:	Native to India and cultivated mainly in India and Guatemala.
Aroma:	Lemony, sweet, strong, sherbet-like, grassy, citrus.
Colour:	Yellow to amber.

Principal properties and indications – keywords

- Astringent
- Refreshing
- Revitalizing
- Tonic

Circulatory system

- ▶ *Excellent for stimulating the circulation.*
- ▶ *Valuable for the immune system, speeding up recovery time after debilitating illnesses such as glandular fever and ME.*
- ▶ *Prevents illnesses from occurring.*

Digestive system

- ▶ *Stimulates the appetite and useful for colitis, flatulence and difficult digestion.*

Genito-urinary system

- ▶ *Very useful after childbirth for aiding postnatal recovery and promoting the flow of breast milk.*
- ▶ *Useful for fluid retention.*

Muscles/joints
▶ *Excellent for improving muscle tone.*
▶ *Relieves tired, achy legs and eliminates lactic acid.*
▶ *Recommended for sports injuries, sprains and bruises.*

Nervous system
▶ *Refreshing and revitalizing for the mind.*
▶ *Banishes apathy and lethargy and lifts depression.*
▶ *Indicated for nervous exhaustion.*

Skin
▶ *A tonic for the skin.*
▶ *Helpful for open pores, excessive perspiration, acne, loose skin after dieting and cellulite.*
▶ *Useful for infectious skin diseases such as scabies and measles.*
▶ *Excellent for fungal infections such as athlete's foot.*
▶ *Highly effective as an insect repellent.*

Effects on spirit
▶ *Uplifting for the spirit, encouraging change and growth.*

Special precautions
▶ *Do not use on babies and young children.*
▶ *Take care with hypersensitive skin.*

Insight
Use lemongrass to spur you into action! Great for that Monday morning feeling or to combat mental fatigue and nervous exhaustion at the end of a long hard day.

LIME

Latin name:	*Citrus aurantifolia*
Family:	*Rutaceae*
Method of extraction:	Cold expression of the peel of the unripe fruit. There is also a distilled lime oil but the aroma is inferior.
Principal constituents:	Limonene, pinene, sabinene, linalool.

Origin:	Native to Asia and cultivated mostly in the USA, Italy, Peru, Mexico and West Indies.
Aroma:	Refreshing, tangy, fruity, citrus.
Colour:	Yellowish-green to olive green.

Principal properties and indications – keywords
- Refreshing
- Revitalizing
- Uplifting

Circulatory system
▶ *Excellent for improving the circulation.*
▶ *Stimulates the lymphatic system.*
▶ *Good immune booster.*
▶ *Helps anaemia.*

Digestive system
▶ *Digestive tonic.*
▶ *Stimulates a poor appetite.*
▶ *Relieves heartburn and indigestion.*

Muscles/joints
▶ *Beneficial for arthritis, gout and rheumatism.*

Nervous system
▶ *Uplifting for those who are depressed or mentally run down.*
▶ *Recommended for apathy and lethargy.*

Respiratory system
▶ *A most pleasant gargle for sore throats.*
▶ *Useful for asthma, bronchitis, catarrh, colds, coughs and flu.*

Skin
▶ *Recommended for acne, boils, chilblains, cellulite, cuts and wounds, oily skin, mouth ulcers, warts and verrucae.*

Effects on spirit
▶ *Uplifts and enlivens the spirit.*

Special precautions
▶ *Avoid strong sunlight immediately after treatment.*

....

Insight

If you feel run down and in need of a tonic it's time to reach for essential oil of lime. Use in your bath to pick you up both physically and emotionally.

....

MANDARIN

Latin name:	*Citrus reticulata*
Family:	*Rutaceae*
Method of extraction:	Cold expression of the peel of the fruit.
Principal constituents:	Limonene, terpenene, myrcene, cymene.
Origin:	Native to China and cultivated mainly in Southern Europe, North Africa and the Americas.
Aroma:	Sweet, floral, tangy.
Colour:	Yellowish-orange.

Principal properties and indications – keywords

- Balancing
- Joyful
- Revitalizing
- Uplifting
- Tonic

Circulatory system
▶ *Tonic for the circulation.*
▶ *Boosts the immune system.*

Digestive system
▶ *Gentle, calming tonic for the digestive system, relieving flatulence and diarrhoea.*
▶ *Useful for stimulating a poor appetite following illness.*
▶ *Good for the liver and gall bladder.*

Nervous system
▶ *Excellent for stress-related disorders.*
▶ *Uplifting, relieving depression and anxiety.*
▶ *Engenders feelings of joy and hopefulness.*

Skin
▶ *Recommended for the prevention of stretch marks and reduction of scarring.*
▶ *Tonic for the skin.*
▶ *Helpful for oily skin and acne.*

Effects on spirit
▶ *Encourages feelings of spiritual happiness.*

Special precautions
▶ *Avoid strong sunlight immediately after treatment.*

Insight
Mandarin is a very gentle oil, therapeutic for young children, in pregnancy and for people who are frail or elderly.

MARJORAM (SWEET)

Latin name:	*Origanum marjorana*
Family:	*Lamiaceae* (or *Labiatae*)
Method of extraction:	Steam distillation of the leaves and flowering tops.
Principal constituents:	Terpinene, terpineol, myrcene, linalool, sabinene, cymene, geranyl acetate.
Origin:	Native to the Mediterranean area. Cultivated mainly in France, Egypt, Germany and Eastern Europe.
Aroma:	Sweet, warming, woody, camphoraceous.
Colour:	Pale yellow to light amber.

Principal properties and indications – keywords
- Calming
- Digestive
- Pain-relieving
- Sedative
- Warming

Circulatory system
▶ *Excellent oil for improving the circulation and relieving chilblains.*
▶ *Regulates the heart and reduces high blood pressure.*

Digestive system
▶ *Recommended for relieving constipation, diarrhoea, flatulence, indigestion, stomach cramps and ulcers.*

Genito-urinary system
▶ *Useful for alleviating painful and irregular menstruation.*
▶ *Helps to quell excessive sexual impulses.*

Muscles/joints
▶ *Very effective for aches and pains, arthritis, rheumatism, sprains and strains.*
▶ *Alleviates pain, coldness and stiffness.*

Nervous system
▶ *Exerts a warming and comforting effect on the emotions easing grief, sadness and depression.*
▶ *Recommended for all states of anxiety.*
▶ *Useful for those individuals who are unable to sit still.*

Respiratory system
▶ *Helpful for colds and flu as an inhalation or chest rub.*
▶ *Effective for coughs.*
▶ *Relieves catarrh and sinusitis.*
▶ *Encourages deeper breathing.*

Effects on spirit
▶ *Excellent for fearful individuals with much agitation and who can find no peace and are constantly searching for the meaning of life.*
▶ *Recommended for detached individuals who find it difficult to be in this world.*

Special precautions
▶ *Avoid during pregnancy (although adverse effects are extremely unlikely).*

....

Insight

This comforting sedative oil is recommended for all states of anxiety. It is particularly useful for the recently bereaved and broken hearted as it instils peace and creates a 'padding' between you and the outside world.

....

MELISSA (LEMON BALM)

Latin name:	*Melissa officinalis*
Family:	*Lamiaceae* (or *Labiatae*)
Method of extraction:	Steam distillation from the leaves and flowering tops.
Principal constituents:	Geranial, neral, caryophyllene.
Origin:	Cultivated in France, Germany, Italy, Spain and Zambia.
Aroma:	Sweet, fresh, lemony.
Colour:	Pale yellow to pale amber.

Principal properties and indications – keywords
- Antidepressant
- Sedative
- Soothing
- Uplifting

Circulatory system
▶ *Beneficial for lowering high blood pressure and palpitations.*
▶ *Regulates the heart.*
▶ *Tonic for the heart.*

Digestive system
▶ *A gentle tonic for the digestive system relieving indigestion, nausea, stomach cramps and liver problems.*
▶ *Stimulates the liver and gall bladder.*

Genito-urinary system

▶ *Regulates the menstrual cycle.*
▶ *Helpful for problems of female infertility.*
▶ *Beneficial for painful periods.*

Nervous system

▶ *Wonderfully soothing for the nerves, dispelling depression, fear, melancholy and insomnia.*
▶ *Recommended for shocks such as bereavement.*
▶ *Counteracts panic attacks and hysteria.*

Respiratory system

▶ *Useful for asthma, bronchitis and coughs, particularly if allergy or stress-related.*

Skin

▶ *Excellent for herpes.*
▶ *Helpful for allergies, wasp and bee stings.*

Effects on spirit

▶ *Uplifting on the spiritual level and helps develop intuition.*

Special precautions

▶ *Melissa is often adulterated with lemon, lemongrass or citronella, therefore take care with hypersensitive skins.*

Insight

On an emotional level melissa banishes negativity, depression and fills one with hope and joy. Melissa is also excellent for herpes. A cream with lemon balm which is sold in Germany is said to reduce the healing time and lengthen the time between attacks.

MYRRH

Latin name:	*Commiphora myrrha*
Family:	*Burseraceae*

Method of extraction:	Steam distillation of the crude myrrh.
Principal constituents:	Curzerene, elemene, myrrh alcohols.
Origin:	Native to North Africa and the Middle East and cultivated in North Africa (especially Somalia), Asia, Yemen and Ethiopia.
Aroma:	Warm, balsamic, medicinal.
Colour:	Pale yellow to reddish-amber.

Principal properties and indications – keywords

- Antiseptic
- Anticatarrhal
- Healing
- Rejuvenating

Digestive system

▶ *Relieves flatulence, indigestion, diarrhoea, irritable bowel syndrome and haemorrhoids.*
▶ *Useful for loss of appetite.*

Genito-urinary system

▶ *A cleanser of the womb, effective for thrush and vaginal discharges of all descriptions.*
▶ *Recommended for scanty and painful menstruation.*

Nervous system

▶ *Helpful for weak-minded individuals who are apathetic, lethargic and difficult to spur into action.*
▶ *Instils calmness and tranquillity.*
▶ *Combats worry and over-thinking.*

Respiratory system

▶ *Highly effective for respiratory problems such as asthma, bronchitis, catarrh and coughs.*
▶ *Dries up mucus.*
▶ *Helpful as a gargle for sore throats and loss of voice.*

Skin

▶ *Rejuvenates mature and wrinkled skin.*
▶ *Heals cracked, chapped and weepy skin.*

- ▶ Combats fungal infections such as athlete's foot.
- ▶ Beneficial for wounds that are slow to heal.

Effects on spirit
- ▶ Beneficial for those who are 'stuck in a rut' and are unable to move on and grow.
- ▶ Helpful for those who see life as a series of negative obstacles.

Special precautions
- ▶ Avoid during pregnancy (although there is no research to support or reject this).

....

Insight
To banish mouth ulcers and also gum infections such as gingivitis try gargling with two drops of myrrh. If you do not like the strong taste I suggest one drop myrrh with one drop lemon or peppermint. Gargle on a regular basis to prevent problems from occurring.

....

MYRTLE

Latin name:	*Myrtus communis*
Family:	*Myrtaceae*
Method of extraction:	Steam distillation from the leaves and twigs and occasionally the sweet-smelling flowers.
Principal constituents:	Cineole, pinene, myrtenyl acetate, limonene.
Origin:	Native to the Mediterranean region and Western Asia. Cultivated in Europe mainly in Tunisia, Corsica, Spain, Morocco, Italy, Yugoslavia and France.
Aroma:	Clear, fresh, sweet, herbaceous, floral.
Colour:	Pale yellow to orangey-yellow.

Principal properties and indications – keywords
- Balancing
- Gentle
- Sedative yet uplifting

Circulatory system
▶ *Stimulates the circulatory and immune systems.*

Digestive system
▶ *Calming for the digestive system and therefore helpful for diarrhoea and flatulence.*

Genito-urinary system
▶ *Good for cystitis and other infections.*
▶ *A tonic for the womb.*

Nervous system
▶ *Relieves stress and tension.*
▶ *Reduces anger and frustration.*
▶ *Recommended for individuals with addictive or self-destructive behaviour.*

Respiratory system
▶ *Excellent for the respiratory system.*
▶ *Combats respiratory infections and coughs and colds.*
▶ *Useful for sinusitis and catarrh.*

Skin
▶ *Useful for acne and oily skin.*
▶ *Helpful for psoriasis and eczema.*
▶ *Excellent tonic for the skin.*
▶ *Recommended for head lice.*
▶ *Regenerates mature skin.*

Effects on spirit
▶ *Lifts the spirits and opens up the heart.*
▶ *Restores faith in the Divine.*

Special precautions
▶ *None.*

Insight

I recommend myrtle for children as a chest rub. It is very gentle and will help to combat infection, expel mucus and induce relaxation. Use two drops diluted in 10 ml carrier oil for a child. For a baby, one drop on a piece of cotton wool placed at the bottom of the cot will help baby to breathe more easily.

NEROLI (ORANGE BLOSSOM)

Latin name:	*Citrus aurantium* var. *amara*
Family:	*Rutaceae*
Method of extraction:	Steam distillation/solvent extraction of the freshly picked flowers.
Principal constituents:	Linalool, linalyl acetate, limonene, geraniol, nerol.
Origin:	Native to Asia. Cultivated in Italy, Morocco, Tunisia and France.
Aroma:	Fresh, floral, haunting, refreshing, light.
Colour:	Pale yellow.

Principal properties and indications – keywords
- Antidepressant
- Aphrodisiac
- Sedative
- Stress-relieving

Circulatory system
▶ *Excellent for high blood pressure, palpitations, false angina and nervous heart conditions.*
▶ *Helpful for varicose veins.*

Digestive system
▶ *Highly effective for colitis, chronic diarrhoea and nervous indigestion.*

Genito-urinary system
▶ *Useful for the menopause and PMS.*

Nervous system
▶ *Valuable for all nervous problems, chronic and short-term anxiety and panic attacks.*

- ▶ *Lifts depression and instils a feeling of euphoria.*
- ▶ *Relieves insomnia.*
- ▶ *Its aphrodisiacal properties make it ideal for sexual problems such as impotence and frigidity caused by tension and apprehension.*

Skin
- ▶ *Wonderful oil for all types of skin.*
- ▶ *Encourages the regeneration of skin cells and works wonders for mature skins.*
- ▶ *Recommended for preventing stretch marks and reducing scars.*
- ▶ *Ideal for sensitive skins.*

Effects on spirit
- ▶ *Puts us in touch with our higher selves.*
- ▶ *Brings peace and tranquillity to a troubled spirit, and for those who repeatedly make the same mistakes in life.*

Special precautions
- ▶ *None.*

Insight

Neroli is one of the most beautiful and effective oils for treating stress. It is an expensive oil but worth the investment. Neroli is also a renowned aphrodisiac – why not try sprinkling a few drops on your bed linen?

NIAOULI

Latin name:	*Melaleuca viridiflora/quinquenervia*
Family:	*Myrtaceae*
Method of extraction:	Steam distillation from the leaves and young twigs.
Principal constituents:	Cineole, limonene, pinene, terpineol.
Origin:	Native to Australia. The majority of the oil is produced in Australia, New Caledonia and Madagascar.

| Aroma: | Sweet, fresh, clear, strong, penetrating aroma. |
| Colour: | Virtually colourless to pale yellow. |

Principal properties and indications – keywords

- Clarifying
- Immuno-boosting
- Pain relieving
- Stimulating

Circulatory system

▶ *Stimulates the circulation.*

▶ *Boosts the immune system.*

Digestive system

▶ *Reduces pain and spasms in the digestive system and helps combat diarrhoea.*

Genito-urinary system

▶ *Relieves cystitis, other urinary infections and discharges.*

▶ *Useful for painful, scanty and irregular menstruation.*

Muscles/joints

▶ *Beneficial for all muscular aches and pains.*

▶ *Good for rheumatism and arthritis.*

Nervous system

▶ *Aids concentration and clears the head.*

Respiratory system

▶ *Excellent for all respiratory problems including asthma, bronchitis, catarrh, coughs, colds and flu.*

▶ *Useful as a gargle for sore throats.*

Skin

▶ *Combats acne, spots and oily skin.*

▶ *Soothes burns.*

▶ *Heals cuts and wounds.*

Effects on spirit

▶ *Purifies the aura.*

Special precautions
▶ *None.*

Insight
Niaouli is one of my favourite oils for a sore throat. Put one drop of niaouli and one drop lemon in a glass of warm water and gargle several times a day to soothe a sore throat.

PALMAROSA

Latin name:	*Cymbopogon martinii*
Family:	*Gramineae* (or *Poaceae*)
Method of extraction:	Steam distillation of the fresh or dried grass.
Principal constituents:	Geraniol, linalool, geranyl acetate.
Origin:	Native to India. Cultivated also in Madagascar, Brazil, the Comoro Islands and Indonesia.
Aroma:	Sweet, rosy, floral.
Colour:	Pale yellow to yellowish-green.

Principal properties and indications – keywords
• Rejuvenating   • Uplifting
• Tonic

Digestive system
▶ *Stimulates the appetite and is useful as a tonic for convalescence.*
▶ *Beneficial for anorexia.*

Genito-urinary system
▶ *Recommended as a uterine tonic and for assisting with childbirth.*
▶ *Useful for cystitis.*

Muscles/joints
▶ *Excellent for relieving stiff muscles and joints, particularly following exercise.*

Nervous system
▶ *Releases stress and tension.*
▶ *Calming and uplifting.*
▶ *Raises self-esteem.*
▶ *Excellent for nervous exhaustion and as a tonic for the nerves.*

Skin
▶ *Renowned for its beneficial effects on the skin.*
▶ *Useful for dry and cracked skin as well as acne since it regulates the production of sebum.*
▶ *Beneficial for mature skin and wrinkles as it aids cellular regeneration.*
▶ *Helps both dry and wet eczema.*

Effects on spirit
▶ *Excellent for a restless spirit.*

Special precautions
▶ *None.*

Insight
The sweet rosy aroma of palmarosa is perfect for relaxing in the bath to soothe away the stresses and strains of a hard day. I suggest three drops of palmarosa and three drops of geranium to restore peace and harmony.

PATCHOULI

Latin name:	*Pogostemon patchouli/cablin*
Family:	*Lamiaceae (*or *Labiatae)*
Method of extraction:	Steam distillation of dried and fermented leaves.
Principal constituents:	Patchoulol, pogostol, patchoulene.
Origin:	Native to Malaysia. Cultivated in Indonesia, India and China.
Aroma:	Sweet, earthy, musky.
Colour:	Dark amber to brownish-coloured.

Principal properties and indications – keywords
- Antidepressant
- Healing
- Hypnotizing
- Rejuvenating
- Soothing

Digestive system
▶ *Curbs the appetite and is useful for those who are trying to lose weight.*
▶ *Useful for relieving constipation, diarrhoea and irritable bowel syndrome.*
▶ *Tones the colon and relieves bloatedness.*

Nervous system
▶ *Popular in the 1960s possibly due to its ability to instil peace, calm and love while at the same time helping to clarify problems.*
▶ *Beneficial for all stress-related problems and sexual problems.*
▶ *Lifts depression.*

Skin
▶ *Encourages the regeneration of skin cells and is recommended for mature skin and scar tissue.*
▶ *Heals chapped and cracked skin and soothes and cools down skin redness.*
▶ *Tones up loose skin after dieting.*
▶ *Useful for fungal infections such as athlete's foot and allergies such as eczema.*

Effects on spirit
▶ *Exerts a grounding effect on those who feel detached from their bodies.*

Special precautions
▶ *None.*

Insight

The musky aroma of patchouli acts as a powerful aphrodisiac. To stimulate sexual desire sprinkle a few drops in an oil burner and allow the sensual aroma to diffuse into the atmosphere.

PEPPERMINT

Latin name:	*Mentha piperita*
Family:	*Lamiaceae* (or *Labiatae*)
Method of extraction:	Steam distillation of the leaves and flowering tops.
Principal constituents:	Menthol, menthone.
Origin:	Native to the Mediterranean and Western Asia and produced mostly in the USA.
Aroma:	Cool, piercing, menthol, minty.
Colour:	Pale yellow.

Principal properties and indications – keywords

- Cooling
- Digestive
- Pain relieving
- Stimulating
- Tonic

Digestive system
- ▶ *Recommended for all digestive problems, alleviating nausea and travel sickness.*
- ▶ *Useful for diarrhoea, constipation, indigestion and flatulence.*
- ▶ *Excellent for pain relief.*

Muscles/joints
- ▶ *Favourable for general pain relief relieving muscular aches, arthritis, neuralgia and rheumatism. One drop in a glass of water may be taken instead of aspirin.*
- ▶ *Exerts a cooling and anaesthetic action when used as a compress on headaches and migraine.*

Nervous system
- ▶ *Stimulates the mind, eliminating mental fatigue and encouraging concentration.*
- ▶ *Recommended in times of crisis as peppermint strengthens yet numbs the nerves.*

Respiratory system
▶ *Beneficial for asthma (especially food related), bronchitis, colds, coughs and flu.*

Skin
▶ *Cools down sunburn and relieves itching and inflammation.*
▶ *Helpful for toxic, congested skin and acne.*
▶ *Useful for infectious skin conditions such as ringworm and scabies.*

Effects on spirit
▶ *Helps to wake up, revive and stimulate the spirit into action.*

Special precautions
▶ *Store away from homoeopathic medications and do not use in conjunction with homoeopathic treatment.*
▶ *Avoid using when breastfeeding as it halts lactation.*
▶ *Take care with sensitive skins (although irritation is rare).*
▶ *Do not use on babies and young children.*

Insight
Peppermint is a great pain reliever and is very cooling. Try a peppermint compress to relieve muscular aches and joint pains. A cold compress of peppermint and lavender placed on the forehead or the back of the neck is a good way to reduce a fever.

PETITGRAIN

Latin name:	*Citrus aurantium* var. *amara*
Family:	*Rutaceae*
Method of extraction:	Steam distillation of the leaves and twigs.
Principal constituents:	Linalyl acetate, linalool.
Origin:	Native to Southern China and Northeast India. Cultivated mainly in France, Paraguay, Italy and Tunisia.
Aroma:	Fresh, floral, bitter-sweet. Reminiscent of neroli.
Colour:	Pale yellow.

Principal properties and indications – keywords

- Antidepressant
- Calming
- Soothing
- Tonic

Circulatory system

▶ *Valuable for stress-related heart problems; it will slow down and regulate a rapid heart beat and dispel palpitations.*

▶ *Stimulates the immune system.*

Digestive system

▶ *Useful for calming the digestive system.*

▶ *Recommended for nervous indigestion, diarrhoea and irritable bowel syndrome.*

Nervous system

▶ *Beneficial for all states of stress and tension.*

▶ *Exerts a calming, balancing effect on the nervous system.*

▶ *Useful in convalescence.*

▶ *Effective for insomnia.*

Skin

▶ *Particularly suitable for oily skin and acne as it exerts a tonic and cleansing action on the skin.*

Effects on spirit

▶ *Opens us up to spiritual levels.*

Special precautions

▶ *None.*

Insight

I think of petitgrain as 'poor man's neroli' as the aroma is so reminiscent of neroli. Whereas neroli is extracted from the flowers (making it much more costly), petitgrain is extracted from the leaves and twigs resulting in a much higher yield. Petitgrain is a reasonably priced oil which you can use on a daily basis to combat stress and induce a wonderful sense of well-being.

PINE

Latin name:	*Pinus sylvestris*
Family:	*Pinaceae*
Method of extraction:	Steam distillation from the pine needles.
Principal constituents:	Pinene, limonene, myrcene, sabinene.
Origin:	Native to Russia, Scandinavia, Finland and the Baltic states. Cultivated all over Europe and the Baltic (especially Central and Southern Europe).
Aroma:	Fresh, forest-like.
Colour:	Colourless to pale yellow.

Principal properties and indications – keywords

- Clearing
- Decongesting
- Enlivening
- Stimulating

Circulatory system

▶ *Useful for poor circulation and for decongesting the lymphatic system.*

▶ *Helps chronic fatigue syndrome.*

Genito-urinary system

▶ *Recommended for conditions such as cystitis as pine has antiseptic properties.*

▶ *Good for fluid retention.*

Muscles/joints

▶ *Combats all muscular aches and pains.*

▶ *Relieves the pain of arthritis and rheumatism.*

▶ *Soothes inflamed joints.*

▶ *Useful after overexertion.*

Nervous system

▶ *Highly effective for alleviating fatigue and nervous exhaustion.*

▶ *Useful for MS and other debilitating conditions.*

Respiratory system

▶ *Excellent for all respiratory disorders.*

▶ *Clears the chest and lungs.*

▶ *Useful for sinus congestion.*

▶ *Helps asthma.*

Effects on spirit

▶ *Pine awakens one's spirit and gives one confidence, courage, strength and patience. It helps one to persevere in the face of adversity and releases guilt.*

Special precautions

▶ *Only use Scots pine oil and not dwarf pine oil which can irritate the skin.*

Insight

The fresh, forest-like aroma of pine is perfect for banishing apathy and lethargy from body and mind. I recommend pine for anyone who is recovering from illness – it will speed up the healing process.

RAVENSARA

Latin name:	*Ravensara aromatica*
Family:	*Lauraceae*
Method of extraction:	Distillation from the foliage.
Principal constituents:	Cineole, sabinene, terpineol.
Origin:	Native to Madagascar and also cultivated in Reunion and Mauritius.
Aroma:	Fresh, clear, penetrating.
Colour:	Colourless.

Principal properties and indications – keywords

- Clearing
- Immuno-boosting
- Stimulating
- Warming

Circulatory system

▶ *Highly recommended for boosting the circulatory and especially the immune system. Ravensara can help the treatment of glandular fever and ME.*

Muscles/joints

▶ *Relieves muscular aches and pains.*
▶ *Useful for overworked muscles.*

Nervous system

▶ *Acts as a tonic for the nervous system and is ideal for nervous exhaustion.*
▶ *Uplifts the mood.*
▶ *Stimulates the brain clearing away stress and tension.*

Respiratory system

▶ *Excellent as a massage rub and as an inhalation due to its antiseptic and antiviral properties.*
▶ *Combats coughs, colds and flu.*
▶ *Effective for sinusitis and all nasal problems.*
▶ *Ideal as a gargle for throat problems.*

Skin

▶ *Recommended for all infectious skin conditions.*
▶ *Use for chickenpox and herpes.*

Effects on spirit

▶ *Encourages you to participate fully in and recognize the joys of life.*
▶ *Allows you to find your soul pathway.*

Special precautions

▶ *None.*

Insight

Ravensara is my favourite oil for boosting the immune system. I always reach for ravensara at the first sign of illness. Gargle with two drops of ravensara in a warm glass of water to ward off coughs and colds.

ROSE

Latin names:	*Rosa damascena (Damask rose/Bulgarian rose/Turkish rose)Rosa centifolia (Cabbage/Moroccan rose)*
Family:	*Rosaceae*
Method of extraction:	Steam distillation of the fresh petals (otto)/ solvent extraction (absolute).
Principal constituents:	Stearoptene, geraniol, nerol, neral, phenylethyl alcohol, citronellol.
Origin:	*Rosa damascena* is mostly cultivated in Bulgaria, Turkey and France. *Rosa centifolia* is produced mainly in Morocco, Tunisia, Italy, France and China.
Aroma:	Sweet, heady, intoxicating, heavenly, rich.
Colour:	Rose otto – virtually colourless and becomes semi-solid at sub-room temperatures. As it is warmed in the hands the oil 'melts'. Rose absolute – yellow to brown-orange.

Principal properties and indications – keywords

- Antidepressant
- Aphrodisiac
- Balancing
- Rejuvenating
- Uplifting

Circulatory system

▶ *Purifying for the blood and is an excellent tonic for the heart.*
▶ *Reduces palpitations.*

Digestive system

▶ *As a cleanser and tonic it is useful for constipation and liver problems.*

Genito-urinary system

▶ *This 'queen' of oils has a remarkable effect on disorders of the female reproductive system.*

- Cleanses, regulates and tones the womb.
- Recommended for PMS and the menopause.
- Renowned as an aphrodisiac and recommended for impotence and frigidity.
- Aids conception and increases the production of semen.

Nervous system
- The exquisite, luxurious aroma has a profound effect on the emotions, alleviating grief, anger, jealousy, resentment, stress and tension.
- Makes a woman feel feminine and positive.
- Recommended for all states of depression.
- Dissolves psychological pain.

Skin
- Excellent for all types of skin, especially dry, mature or sensitive.
- Calms down inflammation and reduces broken thread veins.

Effects on spirit
- Particularly beneficial for a closed heart, encouraging love and compassion.
- Releases past traumas.

Special precautions
- Can be used safely with children. Do not take rose absolute internally.

Insight

Rose, to me, is the scent from heaven. It is my favourite oil for all women's problems – PMT, menopause, all menstrual irregularities and even infertility. Rose instils harmony and positivity and is well worth the investment. Instead of sending a bunch of roses send a bottle of rose oil!

ROSEMARY

Latin name:	Rosmarinus officinalis
Family:	Lamiaceae (or Labiatae)

Method of extraction:	Steam distillation of the flowering tops.
Principal constituents:	Cineole, pinene, borneol, camphor.
Origin:	Native to the Mediterranean. Cultivated in France, Spain and Tunisia.
Aroma:	Clean, strong, slightly camphoraceous, herbaceous.
Colour:	Colourless to pale yellow.

Principal properties and indications – keywords

- Diuretic
- Pain relieving
- Restorative
- Stimulating

Circulatory system

▶ *Excellent for poor circulation and congestion in the lymphatic system.*

▶ *Tonic for the heart, normalizing blood cholesterol levels and arteriosclerosis.*

Digestive system

▶ *Valuable for many digestive complaints, particularly if detoxification is required.*

▶ *Useful for constipation, flatulence, liver congestion, food poisoning and obesity.*

Genito-urinary system

▶ *Recommended for combating fluid retention, discharges, cystitis and painful or scanty menstruation.*

Muscles/joints

▶ *Highly recommended for pain relief in muscles and joints, easing arthritis, rheumatism and stiff, overworked muscles.*

▶ *Useful for poor muscle tone.*

Nervous system

▶ *Activates and enlivens the brain, clearing the head and reducing mental fatigue.*

► *Useful for memory loss and for reviving the senses of smell, speech and hearing.*

Respiratory system
► *Beneficial for asthma, bronchitis, catarrh, colds, flu and whooping cough.*

Skin
► *Use for toxic, congested skin and infectious conditions such as scabies.*
► *Helps abscesses and boils.*
► *Reduces cellulite.*
► *A traditional ingredient of hair care preparations encouraging hair growth, relieving dandruff and combating head lice.*

Effects on spirit
► *Excellent for 'loss' of spirit.*

Special precautions
► *Do not use extensively in the first stages of pregnancy (although side-effects are highly unlikely).*
► *Do not use extensively on epileptics.*

Insight
Rosemary is the great restorer! It awakens the brain, improves the memory and greatly improves energy levels. A marvellous oil to use in your bath/shower first thing in the morning.

ROSEWOOD (BOIS DE ROSE)

Latin name:	*Aniba rosaeodora/Ocotea caudata (Cayenne rosewood)*
Family:	*Lauraceae*
Method of extraction:	Steam distillation of the wood.
Principal constituent:	Linalool.

Origin:	Cultivated in Brazil and Peru. Various misleading articles have encouraged the use of ho wood instead of rosewood for 'environmentally sound' reasons. However, the species is being properly protected and managed with controlled harvesting and farmers are encouraged to replace and expand their plantations. The species is not threatened and therefore it is not necessary to use ho wood oil instead of rosewood oil. The two oils are also different therapeutically.
Aroma:	Sweet, floral, woody.
Colour:	Colourless to pale yellow.

Principal properties and indications – keywords

- Balancing
- Rejuvenating
- Warming

Nervous system

▶ *A marvellous antidepressant, it is a comforting and warming oil which has a balancing effect on the central nervous system.*

▶ *Alleviates stress and anxiety.*

▶ *Clears the mind of clutter.*

▶ *Renowned as an aphrodisiac, it is valuable for frigidity, impotence and other sexual problems.*

Respiratory system

▶ *Beneficial for colds, flu, viruses and throat problems. Rosewood soothes ticklish coughs. It also boosts the immune system.*

Skin

▶ *Suitable for all types of skin – dry, oily, combination or sensitive.*

▶ *Beneficial for treating acne.*

▶ *Highly rejuvenating for the skin, combating prematurely aged skin and wrinkles.*

Effects on spirit
▶ *Recommended for meditation to open up the consciousness.*

Special precautions
▶ *None.*

Insight
I recommend rosewood for rejuvenation. Try a bath with three drops rosewood and three drops rosemary to rejuvenate yourself after a long day at work!

SANDALWOOD

Latin name:	*Santalum album*
Family:	*Santalaceae*
Method of extraction:	Steam distillation from coarsely powdered heartwood and the main roots of the tree.
Principal constituents:	Santalenes, santalols.
Origin:	Native to tropical Asia especially Eastern India. The Indian government has placed certain restrictions on the harvesting of sandalwood which has forced prices up. Other sources of sandalwood now include Indonesia and New Caledonia.
Aroma:	Sweet, warm, woody, lingering.
Colour:	Pale yellow to yellow.

Principal properties and indications – keywords
- Aphrodisiac
- Healing
- Soothing
- Uplifting

Circulatory system
▶ *Tonic for the heart, exerting a sedative yet regulatory effect.*

Genito-urinary system

▶ *Highly effective at alleviating cystitis and vaginal infections of all kinds.*

▶ *Reduces fluid retention.*

Nervous system

▶ *Renowned for its balancing effect on the nervous system, gently soothing away anxiety and tension.*

▶ *Combats insomnia.*

▶ *Recommended as an aphrodisiac and therefore ideal for impotence and frigidity.*

Respiratory system

▶ *Beneficial for chest infections, coughs, bronchitis and sore throats.*

Skin

▶ *Used extensively for all skin complaints, especially dry, cracked and dehydrated skin.*

▶ *Relieves eczema and psoriasis.*

▶ *Recommended as an aftershave when blended with a carrier oil.*

Effects on spirit

▶ *Brings peace and tranquillity to the troubled soul.*

▶ *Recommended for meditation.*

Special precautions

▶ *None.*

Insight

Sandalwood is renowned for its ability to soothe away stress and anxiety. Use it in the bath to gently take away your worries and fears. Sandalwood is one of my favourites for meditation as it creates a sense of profound peace.

TEA TREE

Latin name:	*Melaleuca alternifolia*
Family:	*Myrtaceae*
Method of extraction:	Steam distillation of leaves.
Principal constituents:	Terpinen-4-ol, cineole, terpinene.
Origin:	Native to and cultivated in Australia.
Aroma:	Sharp, strong, medicinal.
Colour:	Pale yellow to almost clear.

Principal properties and indications – keywords

- Antifungal
- Antiseptic
- First aid
- Stimulating

Circulatory system

▶ *Tonic for the heart stimulating the circulation and reducing varicose veins.*

▶ *Highly recommended as an immuno-booster and therefore may help to combat repeated infections, glandular fever and postviral syndrome, myalgia encephalomyelitis (ME).*

Genito-urinary system

▶ *Excellent for cystitis, itching, thrush and vaginal discharges and infections.*

Nervous system

▶ *After an emotional crisis tea tree may be used to ease the shock.*

Respiratory system

▶ *Beneficial for asthma, bronchitis, catarrh, colds, flu, sinusitis, and whooping cough.*

▶ *Ideal as a gargle for throat infections.*

Skin

▶ *A must for every household!*

▶ *Valuable for acne, athlete's foot, boils, burns, cuts, herpes, itching, spots and sweaty or smelly feet.*

- ▶ *May be applied neat to warts and verrucae.*
- ▶ *Recommended for problems with toenails.*
- ▶ *Useful for mouth ulcers and cold sores.*

Effects on spirit
- ▶ *Uplifts the spirit.*
- ▶ *Helps to clear old traumas.*

Special precautions
- ▶ *None. Tea tree is often used neat for first aid purposes.*

Insight

Tea tree is the 'first aid kit' in a bottle. Always take a bottle when travelling for dabbing on cuts and insect bites. Great for warts and verrucae too – apply one drop to the affected area two to three times daily until it disappears.

THYME

Latin name:	*Thymus vulgaris*
Family:	*Lamiaceae* (or *Labiatae*)
Method of extraction:	Steam distillation of the leaves and flowering tops.
Principal constituents:	Thymol, cymene, linalool.
Origin:	Native to the Mediterranean. Cultivated mostly in Europe, Israel and North Africa.
Aroma:	Strong, antiseptic, herbaceous.
Colour:	Pale yellow.

Principal properties and indications – keywords
- Antiseptic
- Stimulant
- Energizing

Circulatory system
- ▶ *Stimulates the circulation and it may be used to raise blood pressure.*
- ▶ *An excellent booster of the immune system.*

- *Benefits chronic fatigue.*
- *Useful for convalescence.*
- *Helpful for anaemia.*

Digestive system
- *Cleanses the digestive system.*
- *Eases abdominal distension, candida and flatulence.*
- *Restores the appetite.*

Genito-urinary system
- *Useful for fluid retention, urinary infections and vaginal discharges.*

Muscles/joints
- *Recommended for sports injuries.*
- *Eases gout, rheumatism and arthritis.*

Nervous system
- *Reviving and energizing oil which stimulates the mind and improves the memory and powers of concentration.*
- *Beneficial for nervous depression.*

Respiratory system
- *Helpful for asthma, bronchitis, catarrh, colds, coughs, sinusitis.*
- *Excellent (as a gargle) for throat, mouth and gum infections.*

Skin
- *Useful for treating head lice and scabies.*
- *Helpful for skin infection.*

Effects on spirit
- *Revives a tired spirit and helps to release blockages caused by past traumas.*

Special precautions
- *Avoid taking during pregnancy.*
- *Take care with sensitive skin.*

▶ *Do not use excessively in cases of high blood pressure.*
▶ *Do not use on babies and young children.*

Insight

If you suffer with low blood pressure thyme is a must-have – sprinkle a couple of drops on to a tissue and inhale several times a day.

VETIVERT

Latin name:	*Andropogon muricatus/ Vetiveria zizaniodes*
Family:	*Gramineae* (or *Poaceae*)
Method of extraction:	Steam distillation of the roots.
Principal constituents:	Vetiverol, vetiverone, vetivene.
Origin:	Native to India and cultivated in India, Indonesia, Comoro Islands, Java and Reunion.
Aroma:	Earthy, smoky, woody aroma, reminiscent of roots and wet soil.
Colour:	Amber to brown.

Principal properties and indications – keywords
- Calming
- Protective
- Tranquillizing

Circulatory system
▶ *Stimulates the circulation.*
▶ *Tonic for the immune system.*

Digestive system
▶ *Useful for a poor appetite.*
▶ *Helpful for IBS.*

Genito-urinary system
▶ *Useful for PMS.*
▶ *Recommended during the menopause.*

Muscles/joints
▶ *Recommended as a muscle relaxant.*
▶ *Alleviates arthritis, rheumatism, cramps, sprains and strains.*

Nervous system
▶ *This 'oil of tranquillity' has a profoundly sedative effect and may be useful for those who are trying to stop taking tranquillizers or other addictive substances.*
▶ *Useful for deep psychological problems and hypochondriacs.*
▶ *Helpful for insomnia.*

Effects on spirit
▶ *Excellent for those who feel out of balance or ungrounded.*
▶ *Useful as a protective shield where individuals are oversensitive.*

Special precautions
▶ *None.*

Insight
The earthy aroma of vetivert, so reminiscent of roots, is perfect for when you feel ungrounded and have that 'out of the body' feeling. Put a drop on a tissue and inhale deeply to bring yourself back to earth.

YARROW

Latin name:	*Achillea millefolium*
Family:	*Asteraceae* (or *Compositae*)
Method of extraction:	Steam distillation from the leaves and flowering heads.
Principal constituents:	Chamazulene, germacrene D, pinene, cineole, sabinene.
Origin:	Cultivated mostly in Germany, Bulgaria, Hungary and Belgium.

Aroma:	Strong, medicinal.
Colour:	Dark to greenish-blue.

Principal properties and indications – keywords

- Anti-inflammatory
- Calming
- Sedative
- Soothing

Circulatory system

▶ *Lowers blood pressure and is a tonic for the circulation.*
▶ *Helpful for arteriosclerosis and varicose veins.*

Genito-urinary system

▶ *Excellent for the female reproductive system.*
▶ *Benefits irregular and scanty menstruation, painful, heavy periods, fibroids and prolapse of the uterus.*
▶ *Recommended for the menopause.*
▶ *Relieves bed-wetting, fluid retention and cystitis.*

Muscles/joints

▶ *Excellent for inflammation.*
▶ *Useful for rheumatoid arthritis, sprains and strains.*

Nervous system

▶ *Exerts a soothing effect on the mind.*
▶ *Helpful for states of anger, impatience and irritability.*

Skin

▶ *Recommended for oily scalp and skin and acne.*
▶ *Useful for inflamed skin conditions such as burns.*
▶ *Beneficial for eczema and psoriasis.*

Effects on spirit

▶ *Valuable for protection.*

Special precautions

▶ *Take care in pregnancy.*
▶ *Do not use on babies and young children.*

> **Insight**
> Yarrow is an excellent oil for soothing inflammation. Try a
> yarrow compress to ease the discomfort of a sprained ankle,
> a pulled muscle, sports injury or arthritis. A compress on the
> abdomen will also help to relieve irritable bowel syndrome.

YLANG YLANG

Latin name:	*Cananga odorata* var. *genuina*
Family:	*Annonaceae*
Method of extraction:	Steam distillation of flowers. There are four grades of ylang ylang. The top grade (first distillation) is ylang ylang extra which has a superior aroma to grades 1, 2 or 3.
Principal constituents:	Linalool, caryophyllene, germacrene D, geranyl acetate, benzyl acetate, benzyl benzoate.
Origin:	Native to tropical Asia. Cultivated mostly in Madagascar, Indonesia, Comoro Islands, Reunion and the Philippines.
Aroma:	Exotic, heady, sweet, floral, seductive.
Colour:	Pale yellow.

Principal properties and indications – keywords
- Antidepressant
- Aphrodisiac
- Euphoric
- Soothing

Circulatory system
▶ *Reduces high blood pressure and has a regulatory effect on the heart.*
▶ *Helpful for palpitations, rapid heartbeat (tachycardia) and rapid breathing (hyperpnoea).*

Nervous system
▶ *Deeply relaxing, releasing anxiety, tension, anger and fear.*
▶ *Uplifts depression and creates a sense of euphoria.*

- ▶ *Restores confidence.*
- ▶ *Relieves insomnia and thoughts that go round and round in the mind.*
- ▶ *Powerful aphrodisiac.*
- ▶ *Recommended for epilepsy.*

Skin
- ▶ *Used extensively for all skin care – both oily and dry skins benefit.*
- ▶ *Promotes hair growth.*

Effects on spirit
- ▶ *Brings peace to the troubled spirit.*

Special precautions
- ▶ *None.*

Insight

Ylang ylang is extremely sensuous and is a powerful aphrodisiac. Light a couple of candles in your bedroom, wait until the wax has slightly melted and then put one or two drops into the melted wax, avoiding the wick.

TEST YOUR KNOWLEDGE

1 Which of the following oils combats catarrh, clears the mind and helps you to study?
   a angelica seed
   b basil
   c benzoin
   d bergamot
   e black pepper

2 Which of these oils is a must-have for babies and children?
   a cajeput
   b cardamom
   c carrot seed
   d chamomile
   e cinnamon

3 If you were going on holiday and you wanted an oil to burn to repel insects which of the following would you take?
   a citronella
   b clary sage
   c coriander
   d cypress
   e eucalyptus

4 Which oil would you choose for digestive problems and travel sickness?
   a fennel
   b frankincense
   c geranium
   d ginger
   e grapefruit

5 Which of the following oils is the most widely used and versatile?
   a hyssop
   b jasmine
   c juniper

d *lavender*
e *lemon*
f *lemongrass*

6 *If you had a mouth ulcer which oil would you gargle with?*
   a *lime*
   b *mandarin*
   c *marjoram*
   d *melissa*
   e *myrrh*

7 *If a child had a chesty cough which oil would you choose?*
   a *myrtle*
   b *neroli*
   c *niaouli*
   d *palmarosa*
   e *patchouli*

8 *Which of the following oils is cooling and effective for pain relief?*
   a *peppermint*
   b *petitgrain*
   c *pine*
   d *ravensara*
   e *rose*

9 *Which oil is a 'first aid kit' in a bottle?*
   a *rosemary*
   b *rosewood*
   c *sandalwood*
   d *tea tree*

10 *If you wanted to create a sensuous and romantic atmosphere which oil would you burn?*
    a *thyme*
    b *vetivert*
    c *yarrow*
    d *ylang ylang*

6

Bach Flower Remedies

In this chapter you will learn:
- *the remedy indications of the 38 Bach Flower Remedies*
- *how to prepare and use the Bach Flower Remedies.*

The action of these Remedies is to raise our vibrations and open up our channels for the reception of the Spiritual Self; to flood our natures with the particular virtue we need, and wash out from us the fault that is causing us harm ... There is no true healing unless there is a change in outlook, peace of mind and inner happiness.

Dr Edward Bach

The Bach Flower Remedies are a simple, safe and natural method of healing. They are becoming increasingly popular and in almost every magazine now 'Rescue Remedy' is being promoted as providing natural relief from stress and tension.

There are 38 Bach Flower Remedies which are all readily available. They aim to restore our balance and enable us to cope with the negative emotions that we experience and the problems that confront us in our everyday life. They are an excellent way to help ease the traumas that we face as we pass through the various stages of our lives.

The Remedies were created by the physician Dr Edward Bach, who became disillusioned with the orthodox idea of treating symptoms with medicines that often had harmful side-effects. He searched the countryside for plants which he instinctively knew would help specific psychological states. Dr Bach was an extremely sensitive and intuitive man and he could 'sense' the remedy that would heal the psychological state. His system of healing is intended to treat the person and deal with the root cause of the problem rather than treating the disease. He firmly believed in the philosophy that a healthy mind ensures a healthy body: 'Take no notice of the disease; think only of the outlook on life of the one in distress.'

Bach began to search for the Remedies that would 'treat the patient not the disease' and discovered 38 flowers which cover the many negative states of mind from which we can suffer. It is well known that persistent worry lowers the body's vitality and its natural resistance to disease so that physical illnesses such as colds, digestive disturbance and other more serious conditions are allowed to develop. If a patient's negative state of mind is treated (fear, depression, hatred, jealousy, guilt and so on) then restoring balance to the mind will restore balance to the body.

The Bach Flower Remedies are a valuable accompaniment to the art of aromatherapy. I firmly believe that every aromatherapist should know how to use them and that every home should have a complete set! There are many parallels that can be drawn between essential oils and Bach Flower Remedies: it is as if they were made for each other. Essential oils are incredibly powerful on an emotional level, often bringing old, unwanted and buried emotions to the surface. The Bach Flower Remedies are absolutely ideal for coping with these states of mind. You will notice that when you read the chapters which concentrate on various conditions, I have indicated which Remedies could be used in combination with the aromatherapy treatments.

I have listed below a description of each of the 38 Remedies. By far the best way to find out and remember what they do is to use them. If you wish to learn more why not try out my *Your Evening Class – Complementary Therapies*.

The 38 healing Remedies – an A–Z

AGRIMONY – Agrimonia eupatoria

Hides mental torture behind a brave face

Remedy indications
For a person who hides their worries, unhappiness and fears
behind a mask of cheeriness. A person who needs this remedy
is troubled, tormented and restless in body and mind and they
suffer inwardly. Often they use their sense of humour to pretend
that there is nothing wrong. In order to ease their inner pain
and to keep up the pretence they will often resort to alcohol
or drugs.

The purpose of this remedy is to allow the person to experience
genuine happiness so that they can be cheerful without pretence.
This remedy works to clear suppressed emotions bringing peace
and tranquillity.

Dr Bach says that Agrimony will bring 'the peace that passeth all
understanding'.

Insight
'It'll be fine! Come on, let's have another drink!'

This person needs Agrimony.

ASPEN – Populus tremula

Vague hidden fears of an unknown origin

Remedy indications
This remedy is recommended for those who experience fear,
apprehension and uneasiness for no known reason. The person
feels terrified that something dreadful is about to happen but has
no idea as to what it might be.

These vague fears may be so pronounced that they haunt the person night and day. The person may sweat and tremble with fear and anguish and will be unable to express their fears to other people; instead they keep them hidden.

The purpose of this remedy is to enable the person to release and to overcome the fears. The individual will develop the quality of fearlessness so that they can face their fears and know that there is no reason to be afraid.

Insight

'I'm afraid but I don't know why – I can't put my finger on it!'

This person needs Aspen.

BEECH – *Fagus sylvatica*

Intolerance of other people's shortcomings

Remedy indications
For a person who is intolerant towards others and finds it difficult to try to understand perceived shortcomings of others. This leads to criticism and such a person will find fault with the way in which other people act and speak. This individual would become easily annoyed by the habits and mannerisms of others who would get on their nerves. Order, discipline, perfection and precision would be important to someone needing this remedy. Intolerance of others and criticism reflects a need for security and is a way of protecting oneself.

The purpose of the remedy is to promote understanding of others and the ability to see beauty and goodness in everyone and everything. One is able to develop a loving acceptance of life in spite of any imperfections.

Insight

'Just pull yourself together. It's your own fault and I've got no sympathy for you.'

This person needs Beech for his/her intolerance of others.

CENTAURY – *Centaurium umbellatum*

Weak-willed/'doormat'

Remedy indications
This remedy is for subservient people who are eager and anxious to please other people. They are unable to stand up for themselves and simply cannot say 'no'. Such people are taken advantage of due to their timid, kind-hearted nature and they become tired and overworked because they always give in to the demands of others. If the weak do not assert themselves then the bullies will become strong.

The purpose of this remedy is to enable the weak-willed to become strong and to assert themselves. A quiet inner strength is developed – one is able to care for others with compassion and wisdom but does not lose one's own individuality and knows when to give and when to say 'no'.

Insight
'People ask me to do things for them and I just can't say no!'

This person needs Centaury.

CERATO – *Ceratostigma willmottiana*

Seeks confirmation from others

Remedy indications
Cerato is for those who lack the confidence within themselves to make their own decisions. Doubting their abilities they constantly seek advice and guidance from others and can be misguided and misled. They are unable to discriminate between what is right and what is wrong and cannot judge what is important and what is superficial. Such individuals will often drain the energy of others by their constant questioning as they try to reach a decision – which they will not stick to anyway.

The purpose of this remedy is to give us the confidence to trust our own intuition, to listen to our soul instead of seeking advice and support from others who may misguide us. We become intuitive and wise and make our own decisions and stick to them.

Insight
'I think I might – but what would you do if you were me?'

This person needs Cerato.

CHERRY PLUM – *Prunus cerasifera*

Fear of losing one's mind

Remedy indications
This remedy is indicated for a person who is desperate that he/she may be on the verge of a nervous breakdown. The mind is so tormented and overstrained that the person fears that they are losing control of their mind and all sense of reason. They fear that they may carry out a dreadful and bizarre action and may even experience impulses to carry out violence and murderous acts, or fear that they may commit suicide.

The purpose of this remedy is to transform the desperate mind into one that is calm and balanced and controlled. We become rational and composed and are able to maintain our calmness and control in all situations.

Insight
'I feel as if I'm losing my mind – I think I'm on the verge of a nervous breakdown.'

This person needs Cherry Plum.

CHESTNUT BUD – *Aesculus hippocastanum*

Inability to learn from one's mistakes

Remedy indications
Chestnut Bud is for those who are unable to learn from their past experiences and who repeat the same mistakes over and over again.

They take a long time to learn the lessons of daily life that are so necessary for our self-development. Such individuals may be repeatedly told or shown something but fail to recognize the pattern and message that is evident.

The purpose of this remedy is to enable us to reflect upon past experiences and learn from our mistakes so that we can go forward into the future, recognizing and avoiding these errors. One wakes up and is in the consciousness of the here and now, watching and learning the lessons of life.

Insight
'I always get myself into the same situations – over and over again.'

This person needs Chestnut Bud.

CHICORY – *Chicorum intybus*

Possessive, selfish, manipulative

Remedy indications
For a person with a possessive love whose caring concern for the welfare of children, relatives and friends becomes selfishly motivated. This results in possessiveness and a desire to manipulate and control the lives of those around them. Such a person will interfere and selfishly demand constant attention and will remind others of their 'duty' towards them. Love does not flow freely and unconditionally from such a person who becomes obsessed with the self, full of self-pity and self-importance. Constant sympathy is sought and if they do not receive the constant attention that they think they deserve they may become manipulative and deceitful.

The purpose of this remedy is to develop selfless care and love for others without expecting anything in return. In Dr Bach's words we 'long to open both our arms and bless all around'. We develop the ability to forget the self and lose our own interests in the service of humanity.

Insight

'I'm your mother. Don't neglect me! I expect you to phone me every day!'

This person needs Chicory.

CLEMATIS – *Clematis vitalba*

Daydreams/lack of interest in the present

Remedy indications

This remedy is for those who are dreamy and drowsy who appear to have no interest in the present. They derive no pleasure from the present, living in the future in the hope of better times ahead. Such a person will often have a vacant look and be inattentive, indifferent and absent-minded. Often they will look listless and only half awake and will doze off at any time as they fantasize about the happier times which might lie ahead.

The purpose of this remedy is to bring us 'down to earth' so that we develop an interest in all things. Instead of escaping into fantasy we develop a strong will to be in life so that we can carry out the work that we are meant to do in this lifetime.

Insight

'I'm sorry, what did you say? I was miles away.'

This person needs Clematis.

CRAB APPLE – *Malus sylvestris*

Cleansing

Remedy indications

Crab Apple is the cleansing remedy and is indicated for a person who is obsessed with cleanliness. Such a person feels unclean and has a sense of self-disgust. They may be ashamed of their physical appearance – often about something of little importance such as a 'big' nose or their cellulite. The disgust they feel may be due to something that they have said or done. People of this nature can become obsessed with tidiness and minute details and their obsessive thoughts of cleanliness and self-hatred rule their lives.

The purpose of this remedy is to clear away the physical poisons as well as mental, emotional or even psychic toxins. We are able to rid ourselves of negativity, develop self-acceptance and self-appreciation and see things in a proper perspective.

Insight

'I hate the way I look, especially my big nose!'

This person needs Crab Apple.

ELM – *Ulmus procera*

Temporarily overwhelmed by responsibilities

Remedy indications
Elm is for a person who is usually capable of dealing with work and personal commitments but who experiences a sudden feeling of being overwhelmed by responsibilities – a temporary despondency. They feel that they have more responsibilities than they can cope with and feel that they will fail. This remedy is often useful for people who are working for the benefit of humanity such as doctors, teachers and healers.

The purpose of this remedy is to give us the strength, courage and conviction to be able to get on with the task in hand despite the difficulties. We develop self belief and faith in our ability to tackle the work before us and feel confident, capable and self-assured.

Insight

'I have so many people who rely on me and sometimes it just gets too much.'

This person needs Elm.

GENTIAN – *Gentiana amarella*

Discouraged/despondent

Remedy indications
It is inevitable as we go through life that we will experience difficulties and setbacks. Gentian is a remedy for those who have a tendency to become easily discouraged and depressed when something goes wrong. The slightest problem or the smallest delay causes doubt that makes such individuals feel disheartened and despondent and even depressed.

The purpose of this remedy is to develop faith and hope in a positive outcome. It enables us not to be affected by setbacks and encourages us to try again and dismiss doubt in the knowledge that there is no failure when we are doing our best, regardless of the result. No task is too big for us to tackle and instead of being discouraged and depressed by our own problems we are able to see the bigger picture.

Insight
'I started exercising last week but I don't feel any better so I'll give up.'

This person needs Gentian.

GORSE – *Ulex europaeus*

Hopelessness/despair

Remedy indications
Gorse is the remedy for those who are experiencing great hopelessness and despair and who have given up the belief that anything more can be done. All hope is lost and they are resigned to the idea that any further treatments will not bring about the slightest improvement. Those who need Gorse have often been ill for a long time and feel they have no hope of ever being well again. In this pessimistic state of mind no treatments will be effective.

The purpose of this remedy is to bring 'sunshine in their lives to drive away the clouds'. It endows us with faith and hope of a recovery. Filled with hope and strengthened conviction that the difficulties can be overcome, we will then be on the way towards a recovery.

Insight

'I've been ill for so long and seen so many doctors and therapists. There's just no point in seeing another one.'

This person needs Gorse.

HEATHER – *Calluna vulgaris*

Self-centredness/self-concern

Remedy indications
A person who needs Heather will be totally obsessed with themselves. They constantly seek companionship from anyone who may be available so that they can talk about their ailments, family problems and their trivia. Such a person is often avoided by others who feel totally drained of energy in their presence. Thus their loneliness and desire to grasp hold of anyone available to listen results in them becoming even more lonely and self-absorbed.

The purpose of Heather is to enable us to become selfless and understanding so that we are able to listen and appreciate that other people have needs too! We are no longer obsessed with our own petty problems and find peace within ourselves.

Insight

'Well here I am again at the doctors. I'm here every week with one health problem or another.'

This person needs Heather.

HOLLY – *Ilex aquifolium*

Hatred/envy

Remedy indications

This remedy is indicated for those who are consumed with envy, jealousy, hatred, suspicion, rage, spitefulness and revenge. If we are filled with such negativity we are also filled with torment, and we will suffer a great deal.

The purpose of this remedy is to drive out the negative thought forms and fill us with the healing vibrations of love and forgiveness. We are able to delight in the success and happiness of others.

Insight

'I just can't stand her! I can't help it – she makes me so jealous.'

This person needs Holly.

HONEYSUCKLE – *Lonicera caprifolium*

Living in the past

Remedy indications

Honeysuckle is the remedy for those who live too much in the past and are so rooted in their memories that they are unable to find joy in the present. It is important that we learn from the past but we should not long to be back there again. We may be nostalgic or have regrets about the past and have a fear of what lies ahead.

The purpose of Honeysuckle is to enable us to enjoy our past memories and to reflect upon them so that we can use the experience and knowledge yet still be able to focus on the present. We can experience joy and fulfilment in the now and progress spiritually.

> ## Insight
> *'Oh it was so much better when I was young. I wish everything was as it was 50 years ago.'*
>
> This person needs Honeysuckle.

HORNBEAM – *Carpinus betulus*

Monday morning feeling

Remedy indications

This remedy is indicated for those who feel weariness at the thought of what lies ahead. We are unable to get going and get on with what needs to be done as we feel tired and lethargic. The 'Monday morning feeling' makes us feel unenthusiastic about the day's activities in front of us. Everything seems like a chore!

The purpose of Hornbeam is to fill us with determination, joy and vitality so that we can get on with all the tasks in hand. We feel a greater zest for life so that we can see each day as a joyful experience rather than as a series of insurmountable problems.

> ## Insight
> *'Whenever I wake up I just can't seem to get myself going.'*
>
> This person needs Hornbeam.

IMPATIENS – *Impatiens glandulifera*

Impatience

Remedy indications

Impatiens was one of the first flower remedies that Dr Bach discovered. It is indicated for irritability, nervous tension and pain. Impatiens is for a person who is quick in thought and action and likes to think ahead and get everything done quickly.

Such a person will find it extremely difficult to be patient with people or situations that are slow and will fidget and feel irritated and on edge. They may finish other people's sentences for them. The Impatiens person prefers to work alone at a fast speed without interference from others.

The purpose of Impatiens is to dissolve impatience and irritability. We are able to become relaxed and more tolerant and gentle towards others.

Insight

'For goodness sake! Why can't this person in front of me get a move on?'

This person needs Impatiens.

LARCH – *Larix decidua*

Lack of confidence

Remedy indications
For people with no self-confidence who do not consider themselves as capable as those around them and therefore tend to take a back seat. They expect failure and feel inferior to others and therefore do not make any effort to succeed.

The purpose of Larch is to take away a fear of failure and to fill us with determination and confidence to take risks and to know that we are capable and can succeed.

Larch is often taken before examinations or when embarking upon new ventures.

Insight

'Oh no. I couldn't possibly go on that course and anyway I wouldn't pass the examination.'

This person needs Larch.

MIMULUS – *Mimulus guttatus*

Fears of known things

Remedy indications

Mimulus is a remedy for nervousness and fear(s) of a known
origin. We harbour many fears – of death, pain, illness, darkness,
flying, heights, ghosts and so forth. Those who need this remedy
will usually keep their fears secret and are often shy and nervous
individuals who blush easily and may feel embarrassed or
uncomfortable in the company of others.

The purpose of this remedy is to make us realize that we have
nothing of which to be afraid. Mimulus fills us with courage
and strength to face our fears and participate fully and trust
in life.

Insight

*'I am going to the dentist next week and I'm frightened of the
injection.'*

This person needs Mimulus.

MUSTARD – *Sinapis arvensis*

Deep black depression that appears for no reason

Remedy indications

This is the remedy for inexplicable depression – a heavy dark
mental cloud that appears for no apparent reason. The gloom
and depression appears suddenly and can be very severe and
debilitating but can lift just as suddenly. It is as if a dark cloud
has overshadowed us and hidden the joys of life. A Mustard
depression may be linked to a past experience in the history of
our soul.

The purpose of Mustard is to make us feel happy and joyful
once again.

....
Insight

'I feel so depressed and down in the dumps but I don't know why.'

This person needs Mustard.
....

OAK – *Quercus robur*

Struggles on despite adversity

Remedy indications

This is the remedy for a person who is naturally brave and will never give up even in the face of adversity. An Oak person would struggle with a chronic illness or a difficult situation and never accept defeat, however much they may be suffering. They are ceaseless in their efforts but there comes a point when their strength begins to dwindle and help is needed to avoid a nervous breakdown.

The purpose of this remedy is to enable us to accept our limitations and to accept that we do need to rest and share our burdens with others.

....
Insight

'I'm really exhausted but I must keep going no matter what!'

This person needs Oak.
....

OLIVE – *Olea europaea*

Mental and physical exhaustion

Remedy indications

Olive is indicated for those who are totally worn out and completely exhausted after a long struggle. This could be due to illness, worry, grief, overwork or a series of difficult problems. It is the remedy for those who are 'burned out' and whose energy reserves have been so depleted that they simply have no more strength left. They tire very easily and have no energy left to enjoy the pleasures of life.

The purpose of Olive is to restore vitality, renew our strength and to replenish our energy so that we can become happy and healthy once again.

Insight

'I'm so completely exhausted. All I want to do is cry.'

This person needs Olive.

PINE – *Pinus sylvestris*

Guilt/self-reproach

Remedy indications
This remedy is indicated for those who blame themselves not only for their own mistakes but also for the mistakes of others and in fact for anything that goes wrong! Even if they are successful they still reproach themselves as they think that they could have done better and achieved more.

Pine is also the remedy for guilt and is tied up with a sense of failing to live up to expectations. We may have been severely told off as children and come to believe that everything was our fault.

The purpose of this remedy is to enable us to see that we are not to blame for everything. We realize that other people also make mistakes and it is not necessary to beat ourselves up as we are all perfect just the way we are.

Insight

'It's entirely my fault. I blame myself.'

This person needs Pine.

RED CHESTNUT – *Aesculus carnea*

Excessive concern and fear for the welfare of others

Remedy indications

This remedy is indicated for those people who project fearful, anxious thoughts onto those around them. They are constantly concerned for the well-being and safety of others and always fear that the worst will happen. If we anticipate misfortune then we will help to create a pattern that will bring it about. Red Chestnut is required when our natural concern for others grows out of proportion and turns into fear and anxiety.

The purpose of this remedy is to calm the mind so that excessive fear for the well-being of loved ones is transferred into a rational concern. It also enables us to remain balanced and calm in any situation.

Insight

'My daughter is out at a party tonight – I won't rest until she is safely in her bed!'

This person needs Red Chestnut.

ROCK ROSE – *Helianthemum nummularium*

Panic/terror/nightmares

Remedy indications

Rock Rose is indicated for the terror, panic and despair that can descend on people in an emergency. Dr Bach described Rock Rose as his rescue remedy to be used in accidents, illnesses and situations where there is seemingly no hope. If the person is unconscious then the remedy can be applied to the lips, temples, wrists or behind the ears.

The purpose of this remedy is to bring peace and calmness to those who are caught up in the emergency. It is to reduce the fear, panic and terror of the moment. Rock Rose may also be used after a terrifying nightmare.

Insight

'Oh no no! I feel I'm having a heart attack. I must call the ambulance.'

This person needs Rock Rose.

ROCK WATER – *Aqua petra*

Self-repression/self-denial

Remedy indications
This remedy is indicated for those who are a hard taskmaster to themselves. These people have high ideals but they have become fanatical about them. They are very strict in the way that they live and they lead a life of self-sacrifice and self-repression, denying themselves the simple joys and pleasures of life. Such individuals try to set the perfect example for others to follow.

The purpose of the remedy is to enable us to adopt a more relaxed approach and to have a flexible mind. We should lead a moral life but should not stifle our enjoyment of life.

Insight

'I go for an hour's walk every day even if it's pouring with rain.'

This person needs Rock Water.

SCLERANTHUS – *Scleranthus annus*

Indecision

Remedy indications
A Scleranthus person is changeable physically, emotionally and mentally. Such people cannot make up their minds. They find it impossible to make decisions – always weighing up one idea against another yet never reaching a conclusion. This indecision can cause mental torment as such individuals are usually quiet

and do not discuss their difficulties with others. Such individuals experience fluctuating moods, such as joy and sadness and optimism and pessimism.

The purpose of this remedy is to enable us to be able to make decisions with calmness and determination.

Insight
'I'm going to town – shall I take the car, the bus or shall I walk? I just can't decide.'

This person needs Scleranthus.

STAR OF BETHLEHEM – *Ornithogalum umbellatum*

Shock

Remedy indications
This remedy enables us to cope with the effects of shock in any form whether it is immediate or delayed. We may have received some serious news, lost someone dear to us or experienced a fright, perhaps following an accident.

Star of Bethlehem comforts and soothes so that our trauma and sorrow is eased.

Insight
'My mother has just died unexpectedly.'

This person needs Star of Bethlehem.

SWEET CHESTNUT – *Castanea sativa*

Anguish/deep despair

Remedy indications
Sweet Chestnut is indicated for feelings of anguish and despair. It is for those moments when our mental torture is so great that

it seems to be unendurable. We have reached the limits of our endurance and can suffer no more. The future looks bleak and holds no hope for us.

The purpose of this remedy is to relieve our deep emotional pain and to reassure us that things can get better. We are able to see that there is a light at the end of the tunnel.

Insight

'I've tried absolutely everything. I'm at my wits' end!'

This person needs Sweet Chestnut.

VERVAIN – *Verbena officinalis*

Over-enthusiasm for a cause/strain and tension due to overwork

Remedy indications
Vervain is the remedy for those who Dr Bach said need 'to realize that the big things in life are done gently and quietly without stress or strain'. Vervain people believe strongly in what they are doing, are highly strung and are incensed by injustice and situations which seem unfair. They try to convert others by imposing their own will and ideas, trying to force people into what is good for them. They tend to overwork, taking on too many tasks at once, and are totally keyed up and unable to relax and often experience insomnia.

The purpose of Vervain is to relieve our stress and tension enabling us to feel peaceful and relaxed and to allow others to have their own opinions and to live their own lives.

Insight

'I work every hour God sends – it's all for a good cause.'

This person needs Vervain.

VINE – Vitis vinifera

Inflexible/domineering

Remedy indications
For a person who is domineering, self-willed, inflexible and strives for power. Vine types are very capable, self-assured and confident of success. They believe that their way is the only way and have no respect for the opinions of others. A Vine person is a natural leader who could become a petty tyrant. A parent ruling the house with a 'rod of iron' is a Vine type.

The purpose of this remedy is to give such a person flexibility in enabling them to put their great qualities to the general good without the need to dominate. Others would be inspired to develop their own potential.

Insight
'How dare you argue with me. What I say goes.'

This person needs Vine.

WALNUT – Juglans regia

Protection from outside influences and life changes

Remedy indications
Walnut is connected with the process of change and the stages of growth. Dr Bach wrote that Walnut is 'the remedy for those who have decided to take a great step forward in life, to break old conventions, to leave old limits and restrictions and start out on a new way'. It helps us to break old patterns and any influences that may be affecting us.

The purpose of this remedy is to enable us to break free and to give us the impetus to move forwards. It is indicated for all changes in life – change of job, a house move, new relationship, divorce or retirement. Walnut is also excellent when biological changes are taking place such as teething, puberty, pregnancy, menopause and during the terminal stages of illness.

Insight

'I just can't get used to my new school.'

This person needs Walnut.

WATER VIOLET – *Hottonia palustris*

Aloof/withdrawing in proud reserve

Remedy indications
For those who like to be alone and tend to isolate themselves, sometimes appearing to be aloof, proud and even superior and condescending. These people seem to be 'different' and will not allow others to interfere in their lives; they bear their problems and sorrows in silence.

The purpose of this remedy is to enable such people to be approachable and to enjoy and appreciate the company of others as well as their own company. Water Violet types can be quiet, gentle, tranquil and wise souls who create an atmosphere of peace and serenity around them and go through life with dignity in a capable and competent manner.

Insight

'I really detest going out. I prefer to stay at home and read my book.'

This person needs Water Violet.

WHITE CHESTNUT – *Aesculus hippocastanum*

Unwanted thoughts/mental arguments

Remedy indications
For those people who cannot prevent unwanted thoughts constantly coming to mind. Worrying thoughts will circle round and round and cause mental torture. These mental arguments take hold and dominate, driving out peace. The sufferer lacks concentration and often does not answer when spoken to. Other symptoms include insomnia, confusion, depression, tiredness and headaches.

The purpose of White Chestnut is to calm, quieten and balance the mind so that we are able to use our powers of thought constructively and can solve problems.

Insight

'The same old arguments just keep going round and round in my head.'

This person needs White Chestnut.

WILD OAT – Bromus ramosus

Finding one's direction/soul purpose/at a crossroads in life

Remedy indications

This remedy is indicated for a person who is unable to find their true calling. Such an individual is usually talented, gifted and ambitious but wants to achieve something really special. However, they are uncertain as to which direction to go in and this leads to dissatisfaction and frustration with life and boredom.

Wild Oat enables us to recognize our potential and to develop it to the full. We become aware of the right path to take in order to live a fulfilled, joyous and useful life.

Insight

'I don't know what I want to do, but I don't want to do this job!'

This person needs Wild Oat.

WILD ROSE – Rosa canina

Resignation/apathy

Remedy indications

For those who have resigned themselves to a situation and make no effort to improve matters. Such people accept their fate whether it be an unhappy home life, a monotonous job or even a chronic illness. There is no effort whatsoever to make any positive changes to life. These individuals lack vitality and are always tired, apathetic and vegetating.

The purpose of this remedy is to reawaken our interest in changing. Motivation, creativity and enthusiasm are restored and this renewed vitality enables us to lead a happy and enriching life.

Insight

'I know my job is boring but I've been doing it for the last 25 years and can't be bothered to look for another one.'

This person needs Wild Rose.

WILLOW – *Salix vitellina*

Resentment/bitterness

Remedy indications
For a person who is filled with resentment, feels hard done by and becomes full of bitterness and self-pity. Such an individual will blame everyone and everything but himself. A Willow type will bear grudges and complain about others' good fortune, acting in a very moody, morose and sulky manner.

The purpose of this remedy is to encourage positivity and optimism. Instead of being a victim, we take responsibility and become master of our fate. We are able to forgive and forget.

Insight

'Oh poor me – I deserve so much better than this.'

This person needs Willow.

RESCUE REMEDY

The well-known Rescue Remedy is a composite of five Flower Remedies, namely: Cherry Plum, Clematis, Impatiens, Rock Rose and Star of Bethlehem. It is used in emergency situations and is even thought to have saved lives although, of course, it cannot replace medical treatment.

Rescue Remedy is useful if we have received a shock of some kind – whenever there is bad news or a family upset. It is recommended whenever we are nervous about a forthcoming event – an exam, a visit to the dentist, an operation, a job interview, making a speech, etc. If we have to work or live under stressful conditions, then Rescue Remedy can be taken in a crisis. I always keep a bottle in my bag to ensure calmness.

Rescue Remedy is not just for humans. Add four drops into your pet's food or drinking water if they have suffered a shock or have been injured. It can also be used for your plants. If a plant, tree or shrub has been re-potted, transported, transplanted or exposed to frost or pests then simply add ten drops of Rescue Remedy into a watering can and use for several days.

Preparation and taking the Remedies

Bach Flower Remedies are completely natural and are extremely safe, producing no harmful side-effects. They may also be taken alongside all medications with no risk of conflict. You cannot overdose on them, and if an inappropriate Remedy is taken it will not cause any ill effects. The Remedies can be taken internally by people of all ages from babies to the elderly. Even pets and plants will benefit.

BY MOUTH

This is the traditional way of taking Bach Flower Remedies. You may take a single Bach Flower Remedy or a combination of Remedies up to a maximum of six. To prepare a Remedy almost fill a 30 ml dropper bottle with pure spring water, add a teaspoon of brandy for preservation purposes and then just add two drops of each of your chosen Remedies. (It is not necessary to add more than two drops – extra drops will not make the Remedy more potent!) Then gently shake the bottle and it is ready for use. Take four drops at least four times a day, either straight on the tongue or in some water. Drops may be added to a baby's bottle or if breastfeeding the mother should take the appropriate Remedies. Use the same number of drops for all ages. However, as you use the Flower Remedies I urge you to be creative.

Insight – Plants

Why not try giving your plants Walnut (as this is the remedy for transition) after they have been replanted or repotted? Fill a 30 ml dropper bottle with pure spring water, top up with a teaspoon of brandy and add two drops of Walnut. Now add four drops from this treatment bottle either to a small plant spray or to a spoonful of water and tip this on to the plant. Repeat this dosage four times a day for best results!

Insight – Animals

Why not try out a remedy on one of your pets or a friend's pet? If the animal is afraid of something – e.g. going to the vet or fireworks – add four drops of Mimulus to the pet's drinking water.

ON THE SKIN

If a person is unable to take the drops orally, the Remedies may be applied to the lips, behind the ears, temples or wrists.

OILS AND CREAMS

Bach Flower Remedies may also be added to oils, creams, lotions and ointments. Add a few drops to a massage oil or an aromatherapy blend to enhance the treatment. For example, if a person was grieving and clinging to the past then the essential oil Frankincense combined with the Bach Flower Remedy Honeysuckle could be used. To help to cope with the effects of change, for example during the menopause, the essential oil Cypress and the Bach Flower Remedy Walnut would make an excellent combination.

BATHS

Another way of using the Bach Flower Remedies is to add them to your bath either on their own or with essential oils. Sprinkle some drops of your chosen Flower Remedy (up to a maximum of seven drops in total) into a bath and soak up your personal prescription. Alternatively, add six drops of essential oil(s) to your bath together with a few drops of your chosen Flower Remedy and enjoy the benefits.

Insight

For a wonderful night-time bath for those who have had a stressful day and cannot switch off their unwanted thoughts try a few drops of Bach Flower Remedy White Chestnut combined with two drops each of the essential oils sandalwood, lavender and juniper.

ROOM SPRAYS

Spraying Bach Flower Remedies into a room either on their own or combined with essential oils is an excellent way to clear the atmosphere of a room.

Insight

To cleanse a room add six drops of the Bach Flower Remedy Crab Apple to a 250 ml plant spray filled with spring water. Add essential oils of juniper and lemon (up to a maximum of 15 drops) if desired. If you want to protect a room from negative energies use the Bach Flower Remedy Walnut either on its own or in combination with essential oils of rosemary, fennel, vetivert or hyssop.

People often ask how long the Remedies take to act but there is no definite answer. The healing could take a few days, a few weeks or even a couple of months. Negative emotions which have developed recently should pass away fairly quickly, whereas deep-rooted problems will take longer to heal.

TEST YOUR KNOWLEDGE

1　*How many Bach Flower Remedies are there – 37 or 38?*

2　*Would a person who is afraid of flying need Aspen or Mimulus?*

3　*Would a person who is impatient and likes to get everything done quickly need Impatiens or Olive?*

4　*Would a person who is very tired need Crab Apple or Olive?*

5　*Would a person who is going through a change in life need Clematis or Walnut?*

6　*Is the cleansing Remedy Chestnut Bud or Crab Apple?*

7　*Would a person who is living in the past need Honeysuckle or Mimulus?*

8　*Would a person who is lacking in confidence need Larch or Centaury?*

7

Aromamassage

In this chapter you will learn:
- *how to set the scene for an aromamassage*
- *the contraindications to an aromatherapy treatment*
- *how to perform a simple aromamassage.*

Massage is a highly therapeutic tool in its own right (see *Get Started in Massage*). When massage is used in combination with the healing qualities of essential oils it constitutes a powerful therapy affecting the physical, emotional and spiritual levels. During an aromatherapy massage emotions are often released alongside the accumulated knots and nodules. The tissues and the nervous system are able to 'remember' both physical and emotional trauma.

Setting the scene

To derive maximum benefit from the treatment it is important to pay attention to the environment in which the aromamassage is to be performed. Careful preparation and the right setting will make a good massage even better. Both the giver and the receiver should feel immediately relaxed. An aromamassage should never be hurried.

> **Insight**
>
> Always ensure that towels, cushions, pillows, mixing bowl
> and oils are on hand so that you do not lose contact and thus
> break the flow of massage.

SOLITUDE AND QUIET

These are vital. Ensure that you choose a time when you will not
be disturbed. Intrusions and distractions are extremely
disconcerting, breaking your concentration and destroying the
flow of your massage movements. Take the telephone off the hook
and tell your friends and family not to enter the treatment room.
You may decide to choose some soothing background music
although this is a matter of personal preference; some will prefer
silence.

CLEANLINESS

This is essential. Always wash your hands before the treatment, as
any stickiness will be instantly obvious to the receiver. Make sure
that your fingernails are short – trim them as far down as possible.
Do not wear any jewellery on your hands. Rings, bracelets and
watches can all scratch the receiver.

WARMTH

The room should be draught-free and warm yet well ventilated.
Nothing will destroy an aromamassage more quickly than physical
coldness: it is impossible to relax when you feel cold. The room
in which you give the aromamassage should be heated prior to
treatment and, as the receiver's body temperature will drop, ensure
that spare towels are at your disposal. Warm your hands if they
feel cold.

> **Insight**
>
> Keep all areas of the receiver's body covered, other than the
> part on which you are working. The receiver should be kept
> warm at all times.

LIGHTING

Soft and subdued lighting will create the ideal atmosphere. Bright lights falling on the receiver's face will hardly induce relaxation and will cause tension around his or her eyes. Candlelight provides the perfect setting, or you may wish to use a tinted bulb.

Insight

Why not add a few drops of essential oil to the warm wax of a candle? Take care to avoid the wick as essential oils are flammable.

COLOUR

The most therapeutic colours to have in the room are pastel shades – pale pink, blue, green or peach decor and towels are perfect for the occasion. Strong colours such as red will tend to create unwanted emotions like anger and restlessness.

CLOTHES

Wear comfortable and loose-fitting clothes as you need to move around easily and the room in which you will be working will be warm. White is the best colour to wear when giving an aromamassage since it will reflect any negativity which is released from the individual being treated.

Wear flat shoes or, even better, go barefoot. The receiver should undress down to whatever level he or she feels comfortable with. Suggest undressing down to the underwear. Point out that areas which are not being worked on will be covered up as this will create a sense of security and trust.

FINISHING TOUCHES

Fresh flowers add a pleasant aroma to the atmosphere, or you can burn incense or essential oils prior to the treatment.

Insight

Crystals may also enhance the environment. Rose quartz relaxes and soothes and amethyst is useful for absorbing negativity. You may put a drop of essential oil on to your crystals. For example put a drop of essential oil of lavender or frankincense on your amethyst or try rose or geranium on rose quartz.

Equipment

AROMAMASSAGE SURFACE

Work on the floor using a firm yet well-padded surface. This will allow you to give an aromamassage whenever you desire. Place a large, thick piece of foam, two or three blankets or a thick duvet on the floor. Use plenty of cushions or pillows during the treatment. When the receiver is lying on his or her back, place one pillow under the head and one under the knees to take the pressure off the back. When the receiver is lying on his or her front, place a pillow under the feet, one under the head and shoulders and one under the abdomen, if desired.

Ensure that you have something to kneel on to avoid sore knees. If you are unfortunate enough to suffer from back or knee problems it may be a good idea to invest in a portable couch. It is far less tiring and makes the receiver's body readily accessible. You could try improvising by using a kitchen table if the height is comfortable for you.

Insight

Do not use a bed as most are far too soft and wide for massage purposes and any pressure applied is absorbed by the mattress. Also a bed will not be the right height for your back.

Your attitude and state of mind

POSTURE

Whether you are working on the floor or at a table, keep your back relaxed yet straight throughout the aromamassage. When standing bend your knees slightly and tuck your bottom in so that your back can work from a secure base (i.e. the pelvis). Allow your thighs to do most of the work – not your back. Remember that it should be as relaxing to give a massage as it is to receive one. With practice you will learn to avoid tensing your muscles so that the healing energy can flow freely through your hands and body. If you do not pay attention to your posture you will become tired quickly. Habits are difficult to break so if you consciously control your posture now instead of slumping it will become automatic later on. Your shoulders, arms and lower back will thus take as little strain as possible. If you are using a couch, stand close to it so that you need to reach as little as possible.

ATTUNEMENT

Your state of mind when giving an aromamassage is vital. The quality and success of a treatment depends upon having a calm state of mind. Do not attempt to give a treatment when you are feeling angry, moody, depressed or unwell. Your negativity will be transmitted. Your complete attention must be devoted to the receiver. If you are worrying about your own problems and your mind is drifting, this will be communicated immediately. Make sure that you are aware of the receiver's breathing and that you are sensitive to his or her reactions. Observe facial expressions and be aware of any tensing up in the muscles.

Insight

Spend time consciously relaxing yourself prior to the treatment and, most importantly, be guided by your own intuition. Take a few deep breaths before the aromamassage

(Contd)

allowing all tension and anxiety to flow out of your body. Breathe in peace and breathe out love. Tune in to the person you are massaging. It may help to work with your eyes closed. Give yourself unselfishly to the massage.

Contraindications

As a general rule, most essential oils are safe provided they are used properly and sensibly. However, please observe the following points at all times.

- ▶ *Do not take internally.*
- ▶ *Do not apply essential oils to the skin undiluted (except for lavender and tea tree for first-aid purposes) as they are far too concentrated and can result in inflammation and allergic reaction.*
- ▶ *Keep oils away from the eyes.*
- ▶ *Keep oils out of reach of children.*
- ▶ *Ensure that the dosage is accurate as too much essential oil can be harmful.*
- ▶ *Purchase only pure essential oils.*
- ▶ *Take care with particularly sensitive skins – it is possible to do a patch test if you are anxious.*
- ▶ *Do not massage where there is a high fever. The body has already raised itself to a high temperature to fight off the infection and does not need the burden of even more toxins to deal with. However, essential oils may be applied on compresses in order to reduce temperature.*
- ▶ *Do not massage the abdomen heavily during pregnancy, especially for the first three months where risk of miscarriage is at its highest. Beware of certain oils throughout pregnancy. Check that there are no special precautions for any of your chosen oils.*
- ▶ *Beware of infectious skin conditions (e.g. scabies), although aromatherapy baths and blended creams are recommended.*
- ▶ *Use only light pressure over severe varicose veins.*

- *Beware of recent scar tissue, open wounds and areas of inflammation.*
- *Beware of unexplained lumps and bumps – always have them investigated by a doctor.*
- *Avoid areas of inflammation (e.g. bursitis – 'housemaid's knee').*
- *Always dilute essential oils when adding them to a baby's or child's bath.*
- *Avoid exposure to strong sunshine or sunbeds immediately after an aromatherapy massage.*
- *Wait a couple of hours after a sauna as the pores are open and the body is still eliminating.*

The treatment

Space does not permit me to describe a complete professional aromatherapy treatment. However, the following sequence will enable you to perform a few simple movements so that you can treat your family and friends. Obviously, if you intend to use aromatherapy professionally then you will need formal training which entails the study of specialized techniques too complicated to describe here. More massage techniques and self-massage are described in detail in another book in the series, *Get Started in Massage*.

THE BACK

Insight

Aromamassage of the back may be used to aid relaxation and release the tense and knotted muscles brought about by factors such as stress, poor posture and a sedentary lifestyle. It can also relieve constipation and menstrual and respiratory problems.

The receiver should lie on his or her front with one pillow under the feet, one under the head, and one under the abdomen if desired.

1 *Start with both hands relaxed at the base of the receiver's back, one hand either side of the spine. Stroke both hands up the back using your bodyweight to apply pressure, spread your hands across the shoulders and then allow them to glide back gently. Repeat this movement as often as you like, to promote deep relaxation.*

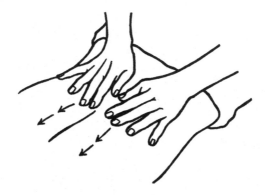

Stroke the back.

2 *Starting at the base of the spine, make small, circular movements with your thumbs until you reach the neck (friction movements). Do not press directly on to the spine itself. Now perform these circular movements around each shoulder blade to loosen the knots and nodules.*

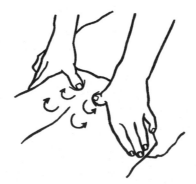

Friction up the back from the base of the spine to the neck.

3 *Repeat step 1.*
4 *Step 4 is performed along the sides of the body and aims to drain away the toxins, both physical and emotional. Place both hands at the base of the spine on the side opposite you. Work up one side of the back pushing the toxins down towards the couch or the floor and gently flick them away. Repeat on the other side.*

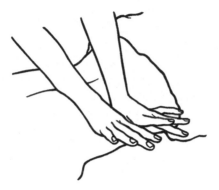

Drain the toxins.

5 *To release tension from the shoulders work across the top of them, alternately picking up and gently squeezing the tense muscles. This movement is called 'wringing' and if you are good at making bread this movement will come easily to you.*

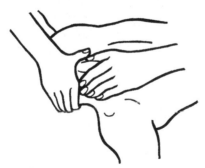

Wring across the tops of the shoulders.

6 *To finish the back repeat the stroking movements as in step 1.*

Insight

Aromamassage of the legs can be used to improve the circulation of the blood and lymph (to cleanse away toxins), relieve cramp and combat fluid retention and it helps alleviate and prevent varicose veins.

1 *Position yourself at the feet of the receiver. Beginning at the ankle stroke up towards the thigh with one hand in front of the other. Use no pressure on the way down.*

2 *To reduce tension from the muscles and to encourage the release of toxins accumulated in the deeper tissues, knead the muscular areas on the calf and thigh. Place both hands flat down and squeeze and pick up the muscles with alternate hands.*

3 *Repeat step 1.*

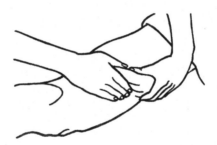

Wring the thigh and calf muscles.

THE FEET

Insight

Regular aromamassage of the feet can dramatically improve the circulation, relieve aches and pains and maintain flexibility and suppleness. It is also wonderfully relaxing and soothing.

1 *Stroke the foot firmly covering the top, sides and sole, working from the ends of the toes towards the ankle. Slide around the ankle bones and glide back to your starting position.*

2 *Support the foot with one hand and use the knuckles of the other hand (lightly clenched fist) to circle firmly over the entire sole of the foot.*

3 *Repeat step 1 as many times as you like.*

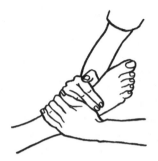

Stroke the foot firmly.

THE ABDOMEN

Insight

Aromamassage of the abdomen is excellent for relieving digestive problems such as bloating and constipation and for menstrual problems such as PMT.

Aromamassage of the abdomen is easy to perform. Position yourself on the right-hand side of the receiver and massage in a clockwise direction, circling around the abdomen with one hand following the other. You are following the direction of the colon.

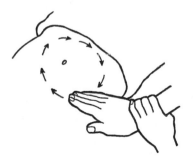

Stroke the abdomen, working in a clockwise direction.

Insight

Aromamassage of the face is deeply relaxing and wonderfully uplifting. It can help to relieve skin problems, headaches, nasal problems such as sinusitis, slow down the ageing process and encourage clarity of thought.

1 *Position yourself at the receiver's head and begin by stroking smoothly across the brow. Stroke outwards across the cheeks and then stroke outwards across the chin.*
2 *Place your thumbs at the centre of the forehead just between the eyebrows, press down and hold for two seconds. Lift your thumbs and place them slightly further out along the brow bone and repeat the pressure. Continue until you have reached the outer corners of the eyes. Work the whole forehead as far as the hairline.*
3 *Repeat step 1.*

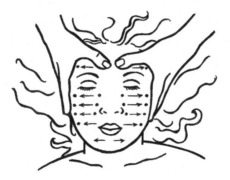

Work across the face in strips using pressure points.

4 *Repeat step 2 on the cheeks and chin.*
5 *Spread out your fingers and thumbs and place the pads on the receiver's scalp. Circle them slowly and firmly, working gradually over the whole of the scalp area.*
6 *To complete your treatment stroke the hair from the roots to the tips and allow your hands to rest gently on the temples.*

TEST YOUR KNOWLEDGE

1 How do you ensure that the receiver is kept warm at all times?

2 What is the best colour to wear when giving a massage?

3 Where do you put the pillows when the receiver is lying on his/her back?

4 Can you massage with undiluted essential oils?

5 What is the effect of friction around the shoulder blades?

6 As you massage the legs is the pressure on the way up or down?

7 Is the abdomen massaged in a clockwise or anticlockwise direction?

8 Name three benefits of aromamassage of the face.

8

Healthy eating

In this chapter you will learn:
- *the basic rules for healthy eating*
- *how to sprout and juice for health.*

Dos and don'ts

Essential oils will help you enormously in your daily life to improve your health and alleviate many common health problems. However, as I stated in the introduction, aromatherapy is a holistic therapy and dietary changes are necessary if true healing is to take place. Space does not allow me to explore dietary advice in any great detail but if you wish to explore nutrition in more detail then please refer to *Teach Yourself Detox*.

> **Insight**
> The ideal diet should include a high proportion of fruit, vegetables and salads. Other foods, such as bread and other starchy foods, meat, cheese, eggs and so on, should form only about 20–30 per cent of your diet as it is these foods which cause problems such as the overproduction of mucus, tension in the nervous system, arthritis, rheumatism, digestive disorders and respiratory problems, etc.

To start you on the right dietary path to health and fitness try to stick to these basic easy-to-follow rules:

DO

▶ *Eat plenty of fresh fruit.*
▶ *Eat more fresh vegetables.*
▶ *Eat more salads.*
▶ *Chew your food thoroughly and slowly in pleasant surroundings.*
▶ *Steam or stir-fry your vegetables – if you boil your vegetables then many of the nutrients are left in the water.*
▶ *Use cold-pressed vegetable oils (such as virgin olive oil) instead of saturated fats which can lead to heart disease, raised blood pressure and cholesterol as well as weight gain.*
▶ *Drink water which is necessary to keep all our bodily functions working, removing waste and preventing constipation. At least six to eight glasses per day is healthy.*
▶ *Have a treat occasionally!*

Insight

A good indication that you are drinking enough water is the colour of your urine which should be a pale yellow colour – not cloudy or dark in colour.

DON'T

▶ *Eat processed foods from cans and packets that contain chemical additives such as colourings and preservatives. Harmful additives can lead to hyperactivity and allergies and have been linked with cancer.*
▶ *Use too much salt which can result in high blood pressure, strokes, heart attacks and waterlogged tissues.*
▶ *Use too much sugar which lacks nourishment and is linked with heart disease, hardening of the arteries, obesity, mood changes, tooth decay and so forth.*
▶ *Eat too much meat, especially red meat which has been linked with heart disease, strokes and cancer. Putrefying waste matter*

remains in the large intestine for long periods, toxifying the body – the average person has three to five kilos of rotting waste matter in the colon. Most meat contains chemicals, antibiotics and growth hormones. If possible eat organically reared meat and increase your fish intake.

▶ *Eat too many dairy foods which can encourage mucus and a whole host of other diseases such as arthritis, colds, allergies, asthma and skin diseases. Do not worry that your teeth will fall out and your bones will collapse as green leafy vegetables and raw nuts and seeds are all excellent sources of calcium.*

▶ *Drink too many cups of tea and coffee and be careful with the word 'decaffeinated' which may indicate that although the caffeine has been removed the chemicals theophylline and theobromine remain which affect humans in a similar way to caffeine! Try to reduce your tea and coffee intake by replacing some with water, herb teas and fruit juices.*

▶ *Drink too much alcohol. In moderation it is fine (especially red wine) but in excess will damage the body.*

▶ *Smoke – cigarettes contain harmful chemicals and damage the heart and lungs.*

Insight

Cigarette smoke contains 2,000 chemicals including nicotine, arsenic, cyanide and cadmium. Smoking damages the heart and lungs, elevates blood pressure, damages the liver and affects the digestion. Try essential oil of clary sage to curb smoking and also Rescue Remedy to help decrease stress levels.

Sprouting for health

Packed with a superb balance of vitamins, minerals, protein, carbohydrates and fat, the seeds of a plant are our finest source of nutrition. But there's something we have to do to them to unlock all of this potential – we have to trigger their growth (germination) into a young plant by soaking them in water for a few days. This process is called sprouting.

THE BENEFITS OF SPROUTING

In an age when most fruit and vegetables are grown in artificially fertilized soils and treated with all manner of chemicals including hormones, fungicides, insecticides and preservatives, seeds sprouted at home in a jar are a trusty, easily accessible source of organically grown nutrition.

Not only do many sprouted foods taste great, but they are also highly health promoting. For starters, as a seed sprouts, the nutrients within increase their concentration in sheer quantum leaps – proteins by about 20 per cent, nucleic acids by 30 per cent, and many vitamins by a staggering 500 per cent!

At the same time, enzymes dormant in seeds spring into life breaking down starch into simple sugars like fructose and sucrose, splitting proteins into amino acids and converting saturated fats into free amino acids. It is also believed that this high enzyme activity stimulates the body's own enzymes into greater activity. Interestingly, when dormant, chickpeas, lentils and mung beans are filled with enzyme inhibitors which not only make them difficult to digest – even when cooked – but can also interfere with our ability to absorb minerals in the food.

Insight

Sprouts make a nutritious addition to salads, sandwiches and soups. You can also fry them gently in olive oil and add them to casseroles or omelettes.

WHAT CAN WE SPROUT?

You might be surprised to hear that we can sprout just about any living vegetation, including beans, legumes, grains, nuts, seeds and even some grasses such as barley grass or wheat grass. However, the most common foods that people sprout are adzuki beans, mung beans, soya beans, chickpeas, oats, lentils, mustard, radish, quinoa, sesame seeds and sunflower seeds. When sprouted, these all make delicious snacks, especially when added to salads with a good dressing.

HOW DO WE SPROUT SEEDS?

The best way to sprout seeds is to buy a sprouter – a three-tiered tray system.

The process involved is as follows:

1 *Choose your seeds – organic are best.*
2 *Place the seeds in a bowl and rinse them thoroughly in water.*
3 *Place them in your sprouter and cover them with cooled, boiled water.*
4 *Leave them overnight in a warm, dark place.*
5 *In the morning, rinse your seeds with fresh water and return them to the warm, dark location.*
6 *Do the same in the evening.*
7 *Repeat steps 5 and 6 until the seeds begin to sprout.*
8 *When the seeds have begun to sprout, place them on a windowsill to get some warmth from the sun.*
9 *The sprouted seeds can now be removed from the sprouter.*
10 *Sprinkle the sprouts onto a salad or a stir-fry, or eat them as a snack in their own right.*

HARVESTING TIMES

The table below is an approximate guide to how long it takes to harvest different seeds.

Seed harvesting time (days)	
Adzuki beans	4–6
Barley	3–4
Chickpea	4–5
Fenugreek	4–5
Flageolet beans	3–5
Green lentils	3–5
Green peas	3–5

Mung beans	2–3
Pumpkin seeds	4–6
Radish	4–5
Rye	3–5
Sunflower seeds	4–6

SPROUTED SALAD RECIPE

It is always nice to use a mixture of sprouts, as in this recipe.

50 g mangetout
50 g sprouted chickpea and mung bean mix
25 g mustard sprouts
1/2 chicory
1/2 bunch of watercress
Optional: 1 container of marinated tofu pieces
Balsamic vinaigrette dressing or olive oil

Wash and dry the mangetout, chicory and watercress. Toss everything in a bowl and mix the balsamic vinaigrette dressing or olive oil with cracked pepper to taste.

Juicing for health

A fresh juice every day can provide you with all the vitamins and minerals you need.

More and more of us understand the importance of eating a diet rich in fruit and vegetables, but if you would like to try an alternative way of getting your vitamins and minerals, why not try juicing? Are you aware of the wonders of juicing and the health benefits you can receive from doing so? There are lots of fantastic recipes and creations that you can put together to suit all tastes, and you can even get the kids involved too! Here are ten very good reasons to try juicing:

1 **Stock up on enzymes** – *juices are very rich in enzymes that help digest your food. A shortage of enzymes means we cannot convert foods into energy or transform carbohydrates, proteins, fats, vitamins and minerals into what we need for healthy tissue such as muscle, bone, skin, and so on.*

2 **Load up on essential nutrients** – *vitamins and minerals are essential for good health. Vitamins fall in to two categories, water-soluble (vitamins B and C) and fat-soluble (vitamins A, D and E). Many factors affect our vitamin status including inadequate diet, digestion problems, over-cooking, canned and processed foods, storage and irradiation. Fresh juicing supplies the vitamins and minerals we need in abundance.*

3 **Boost your vitality** – *juicing is a high vitality 'food' that is very nourishing and revitalizing to the cells. Dr Max Gerson, founder of the Institute for Cancer Treatments, found that his patients tended to recover from degenerative illnesses more quickly when put on a diet made largely from fresh raw juices.*

4 **Eliminate toxins** – *fresh fruit and vegetable juices are a must for all detox diets. Some juices have the ability to rid the body of waste and bacteria and to deep-cleanse the body.*

5 **Get plenty of chlorophyll** – *chlorophyll can be found in abundance in all green plants. It cleanses your digestive system and builds blood cells, making it an all-round great tonic. Alfalfa, wheatgrass, watercress and leafy greens are all high in chlorophyll and are fantastic in juices.*

6 **Reduce your risk of premature disease** – *this can be aided by the antioxidants contained in juices. Beauty, like health, comes from within so what we eat plays a vital role. Antioxidants are thought to be the secret to living longer and looking younger as they 'mop up' harmful molecules known as 'free-radicals'.*

7 **Get your essential amino acids** – *these are the building blocks of protein and are vital in the process of digestion and assimilation of food. Fresh raw juices are rich in amino acids and are in an easily digestible form.*

8 **Balance acid/alkaline levels** – *Western diets tend to be high in animal protein, refined sugar and artificial additives and drugs. All of these cause acidity in the cells, which, in turn, can lead to disease. It is well documented that cancer cells thrive in an acidic environment.*

9 **Aid weight reduction** – *juices are both 'filling' and yet low in calories. They help curb the appetite and are, therefore, an important part of many weight-loss programmes.*

10 **Enjoy all the tastes** – *try to be creative and try some of the recipes below. They all have health benefits and will awaken the taste-buds ... so why not get juicing!*

Insight

For best results use organically grown unsprayed produce. A lemon bath rinse is an excellent way to destroy bacteria, pesticides and agricultural chemicals. Simply fill a large bowl with cold water, add the juice of a freshly squeezed lemon and a small tablespoon of salt. Place your fruit and vegetables into the lemon bath for 5–10 minutes and then rinse thoroughly in cold water.

APPLE, CARROT AND BEETROOT JUICE

1 carrot (unpeeled, topped and tailed)
1 red apple
1 beetroot (skinned and washed, leave the roots and tops on)

This juice will be high in vitamins A, C, calcium, magnesium, potassium and iron.

LEMONADE

1/2 wedge lemon (unwaxed)
2–3 golden delicious apples

Juice and serve over crushed ice. This will be a good cleanser and the lemons will have an alkalizing effect.

POPEYE SPECIAL

1 apple
1 stick of celery (with the leaves)
75 g spinach (fresh young leaves)
1 small bunch watercress
1 small bunch of wheatgrass (if desired)

This will be rich in vitamins A, C, folic acid and riboflavin (B_2).

In the following chapters, which are concerned with disorders that may be improved by aromatherapy, I outline simple dietary changes that can be used alongside your aromatherapy treatments to promote health.

TEST YOUR KNOWLEDGE

1 *How many glasses of water should you drink per day?*

2 *Give two reasons why too much sugar is harmful.*

3 *Name two ways in which sprouts can be incorporated into the diet.*

4 *Is the Western diet usually more acid or more alkaline?*

5 *For best results in juicing what sort of produce should be used?*

9

Circulation

In this chapter you will learn:
* *the causes and effects of the most common circulatory disorders*
* *the orthodox treatment for these conditions*
* *which aromatherapy oils are indicated for each disorder and why*
* *how dietary and lifestyle changes can help*
* *which Bach Flower Remedies to take.*

Anaemia

Anaemia is the most common blood disease and is characterized by a deficiency of the haemoglobin (iron-containing) component of the red blood cells. Since red blood cells carry oxygen from the lungs to the tissues of the body in exchange for carbon dioxide, anaemia can also be thought of as a lack of oxygen being transported to the tissues in appropriate amounts and a build-up of carbon dioxide.

SYMPTOMS

▶ *fatigue, lassitude and a tendency to tire easily*
▶ *shortness of breath especially on exercise*
▶ *dizziness/fainting*
▶ *disturbed vision*
▶ *loss of appetite*
▶ *pallor of the skin*
▶ *palpitations*

- *angina*
- *rapid pulse*
- *ankle oedema (swelling) in severe cases where heart failure develops.*

There are a number of varieties of anaemia, but for the purposes of this book I shall discuss only iron deficiency anaemia. This type of anaemia has three causes:

- *Blood loss as in menstruation and bleeding from the gastrointestinal tract as in ulcers, hiatus hernia and cancer. Even slight losses of blood if they occur over a long period of time can lead to anaemia – 1 ml of blood contains 0.5 mg of iron. Studies in developed countries have found evidence of iron deficiency in 30–50 per cent of the population. Iron deficiency usually develops slowly.*
- *Increased body requirements as in pregnancy and during periods of rapid growth and lactation.*
- *Nutritional deficiency caused by poor diet, ignorance, lack of food or malabsorption.*
- *In addition to the general features of anaemia, iron deficiency is also characterized by a sore, smooth, red tongue, dry, brittle, spoon-shaped nails, 'pins and needles' and difficulties in swallowing.*

TREATMENT

Orthodox treatment
A laboratory analysis of the blood is performed and a course of iron tablets or occasionally iron injections will be recommended. It is vital that the underlying cause is found.

Aromatherapy treatment
The following essential oils are particularly indicated for the treatment of anaemia:

Black pepper is a stimulant of the spleen which is involved in the production of new blood cells. It is also a stimulating and warming oil, in general helping to alleviate the feelings of utter exhaustion always associated with anaemia.

German/Roman chamomile, geranium and **lemon** are useful where the cause of anaemia is found to be menorrhagia (heavy menstrual blood loss). They will help to reduce the heavy bleeding, particularly lemon.

Thyme is also valuable in the treatment of anaemia. It is a powerful stimulant and is widely used when the body is working 'under par'. Thyme is excellent for combating fatigue and lethargy and it also helps to stimulate the appetite which is often so poor where anaemia is present. It also stimulates the production of white corpuscles, thus strengthening the body's resistance to illness.

Baths
Take daily baths using any of the following oils:

▶ **black pepper, carrot seed, chamomile, geranium, lemon, lime, rosemary, thyme.**

Insight
One of my favourite recipes for anaemia for use in the bath is two drops black pepper, two drops German/Roman chamomile and two drops lemon.

Inhalations
Sprinkle a few drops of black pepper, lemon or thyme on a tissue and inhale several times deeply, keeping the eyes shut.

Aromamassage
The following oils may be helpful:

2 drops German/Roman chamomile 1 drop geranium 2 drops lemon	or	2 drops black pepper 2 drops German/ Roman chamomile 1 drop lemon 1 drop thyme	diluted in 15 ml carrier oil

Contraindications

Thyme should be avoided during pregnancy and if the skin is exceptionally sensitive, and should not be used excessively in cases of high blood pressure. **Lemon** should not be applied prior to sunbathing.

BACH FLOWER REMEDIES

The Bach Flower Remedy **Olive** is particularly indicated where the individual feels utterly exhausted and even totally drained to the point of crying.

For feelings of helplessness, despondency, despair and negativity, **Gorse** is strongly recommended.

DIET

A diet high in iron-rich foods is recommended, particularly during menstruation and pregnancy. Foods rich in iron include liver, green leafy vegetables, blackstrap molasses, dried apricots and other dried fruits, alfalfa sprouts, spirulina, wheatgrass, beetroot, lettuce (dark leafy kind) and ginseng.

Insight

A supplement of vitamin C enhances the absorption of iron greatly. At least 1 g of vitamin C daily is indicated. Iron absorption is inhibited by drinking tea and coffee immediately after meals and by antacids. These should, therefore, be reduced or avoided.

Angina pectoris

Angina pectoris is caused by a lack of oxygen reaching the heart muscle, usually as a result of coronary vessel arteriosclerosis. This creates an atheromatous plaque which narrows and eventually blocks the coronary artery, resulting in a decreased blood and oxygen supply to the heart tissue and creating the characteristic pain. Angina is usually brought on by exertion and relieved by rest and nitrate drugs. It is also precipitated by stress, anxiety, emotion and any other situations making demands upon the heart.

SYMPTOMS

- *constricting pain in the centre of the chest often radiating to the left shoulder blade and arm, neck, throat or jaw*
- *dyspnoea (breathing difficulties), nausea, sweating and faintness.*

TREATMENT

Orthodox treatment
Angina requires strict medical supervision. Drug therapy is indicated and if this fails, coronary artery bypass surgery may be carried out.

Aromatherapy treatment
The aims of aromatherapy are to reduce stress and improve the circulation.

Baths
Take daily baths with the addition of six drops of any of the following oils:

- benzoin, black pepper, geranium, ginger, marjoram *and* rosemary *will help to improve the circulation*
- bergamot, German/Roman chamomile, clary sage, frankincense, jasmine, neroli, rose, sandalwood, vetivert *and* ylang ylang *will alleviate tension.*

> ## Insight
> An excellent combination of oils to use in the bath is two drops bergamot, two drops frankincense and two drops ginger.

Inhalations
Put a few drops of **lavender** on a tissue and inhale deeply, keeping the eyes closed. This will help to reduce stress, anxiety and the panic related to an attack of angina.

Aromamassage
Regular massage treatment is of enormous benefit in cardiac conditions. Massage is advisable at least once a month. The following formulae are recommended or you may create your own formulae choosing from the list:

1 drop bergamot 1 drop clary sage 1 drop ylang ylang	} or	1 drop frankincense 1 drop geranium 1 drop marjoram	} diluted in 10 ml carrier oil
1 drop benzoin 1 drop ginger 1 drop neroli	} or	1 drop bergamot 1 drop ginger 1 drop neroli	} diluted in 10 ml carrier oil

Contraindications
Avoid **marjoram** in pregnancy, although adverse effects are highly unlikely. Avoid **bergamot** prior to sunbathing.

BACH FLOWER REMEDIES

The Bach Flower Remedy **Impatiens** is valuable for alleviating states of anxiety, impatience and irritability. **White Chestnut** is excellent for those whose minds are constantly occupied with persistent worrying thoughts. **Star of Bethlehem** will help to take away the effects of shock and trauma which can precipitate or occur after an attack. **Mimulus** can be taken by those who are fearful that another angina attack may occur.

DIET

It is essential to eat a healthy diet if angina has been diagnosed. Avoid junk food as much as possible since it contains high levels of sugar and salt. Avoid all fried foods – try to steam or grill.

Eat plenty of fresh fruit and vegetables. Saturated animal fats such as lard, butter and hydrogenated vegetable oil have been linked with a high risk of heart disease and cholesterol levels. Extra virgin olive oil is excellent and it is interesting to note that in Mediterranean countries, where enormous amounts of olive oil are consumed, the incidence of angina is low. Essential fatty acids are thought to prevent heart disease. They are present in oily fish such as mackerel, salmon, sardines and herring as well as in seed oils (flax and hemp) and vegetable oils. Dietary fibre also appears to protect the heart, although more research is needed. It is present in all plant foods including cereals (especially oats) and vegetables, pulses, fruits, nuts and seeds.

Insight

Garlic is excellent for thinning the blood and it should be eaten raw whenever possible. Ideally eat one or two raw cloves daily as cooking decreases the nutritional value. After eating garlic chew fresh parsley to sweeten the breath.

Supplements which may be useful include coenzyme Q10 (CoQ10) which is thought to enhance energy production within the heart. Studies show that CoQ10 deficiency is common in patients with heart disease. Magnesium reduces spasms in the coronary arteries and improves heart function. Garlic capsules are recommended (although raw garlic is preferable). L-arginine amino acid (5000 mg daily) improves blood circulation and facilitates vasodilation. Eating cantaloupe melon and pineapple has also proved to be beneficial to help alleviate attacks due to their vitamin C and bromelain content.

Obviously you should not smoke, and if you are obese then you should try to lose weight slowly and sensibly. Gentle, regular physical exercise is vital for a healthy heart so try to take a 20 minute walk daily.

Hawthorn extracts are also of great value to sufferers of angina and other heart diseases. Experimental studies reveal that hawthorn dilates coronary blood vessels thus improving the blood and oxygen supply to the heart.

High blood pressure (hypertension)

The World Health Organization defines high blood pressure as a systolic pressure greater than 160 and a diastolic pressure greater than 95. Currently 90–95 per cent of all diagnosed hypertension is termed 'essential hypertension' (i.e. the underlying mechanism is unknown). In the other 5–10 per cent the hypertension is secondary to another disease (e.g. kidney disease, drugs, pregnancies, hormonal problems).

Severe hypertension is a serious disorder (systolic pressure greater than 220 or diastolic pressure greater than 140), requiring emergency treatment before heart or kidney failure, cerebral haemorrhage or fits occur. High blood pressure is a fairly common disorder and the incidence increases with age.

SYMPTOMS

- *headaches*
- *visual disturbance*
- *ringing in the ears*
- *breathlessness and/or chest pain.*

TREATMENT

Orthodox treatment
Drug therapy involves the use of diuretics and/or beta-adrenergic blocking drugs and vasodilators. Antihypertensive medications are among the most widely prescribed. Unfortunately there can be side-effects.

All clients with hypertension should change both their diet and lifestyle. If the guidelines suggested are followed, most individuals will see a reduction in blood pressure.

If hypertension is not controlled then it can lead to hardening of the arteries (atheroma), heart failure, coronary disease and strokes.

Aromatherapy treatment

Aromatherapy can have a profound effect on blood pressure, although it is essential that dietary and lifestyle changes are also made. Essential oils which encourage deep relaxation and stress reduction are particularly valuable.

Baths

Daily baths with essential oils added are highly therapeutic. Particularly useful essential oils include **chamomile, clary sage, frankincense, geranium, juniper, lavender, lemon, marjoram, melissa, neroli, rose, yarrow** and **ylang ylang**. Suggested combinations are:

2 drops lavender 2 drops marjoram 2 drops ylang ylang	or	2 drops clary sage 2 drops frankincense 2 drops marjoram	or	2 drops German/Roman chamomile 2 drops geranium 2 drops rose

If a cleansing, detoxifying action is required, for instance when dietary changes are being implemented, use two drops **fennel**, two drops **juniper** and two drops **lemon**.

Inhalations

Sprinkle a few drops of lavender or two drops lavender and two drops marjoram on a tissue and inhale deeply several times a day.

Aromamassage

Aromamassage once a week is highly recommended for reducing blood pressure.

Insight

If aromamassage is performed at regular intervals the effects are quite remarkable and blood pressure may be lowered for several days after a treatment. The massage should be gentle and soothing, always in the direction of the heart.

Suggested formulae:

$\left.\begin{array}{l} \text{1 drop clary sage} \\ \text{1 drop frankincense} \\ \text{1 drop lavender} \end{array}\right\}$ or $\left.\begin{array}{l} \text{1 drop marjoram} \\ \text{1 drop neroli} \\ \text{1 drop ylang ylang} \end{array}\right\}$ diluted in 10 ml of carrier oil

For a detoxifying aromatherapy treatment:

$\left.\begin{array}{l} \text{2 drops juniper berry} \\ \text{1 drop lemon} \end{array}\right\}$ diluted in 10 ml of carrier oil

Contraindications

Fennel should be avoided in pregnancy and should be used sparingly by epileptics. **Marjoram** should be avoided in pregnancy, although an adverse reaction is highly unlikely. Avoid strong sunlight after the application of **lemon**.

BACH FLOWER REMEDIES

Remedies for stress relief include **Rescue Remedy, Impatiens** and **Vervain**. For those individuals who fail time and time again to learn their lesson that stress is no good for them, **Chestnut Bud** is an excellent choice.

DIET

The diet should be low in salt, sugar and saturated fats as the effects of these substances on blood pressure are well documented. As the public has become aware of the dangers of salt, purchases of table salt have decreased but it is also important to look for hidden salt in processed and prepared foods. Sugar is also hidden in many foods. Increasing dietary linoleic acid as found in vegetable oils in Mediterranean countries, where the incidence of hypertension is lower, has an enormous hypotensive action. Fatty red meat can also cause blood pressure to rise.

A whole food diet emphasizing fruit and vegetables and garlic is recommended, with plenty of dietary fibre, particularly oat fibre.

The link between obesity and hypertension is well researched, and weight reduction will cause a substantial reduction in blood pressure. Weight reduction is probably more effective than taking antihypertensive drugs.

Caffeine, alcohol and smoking should also be eliminated from the diet as far as possible. Evidence reveals that 200 mg of caffeine (approximately three cups of black coffee) produces a temporary rise in blood pressure. Too much alcohol produces a significant rise in blood pressure in some individuals. It is well documented that smoking contributes to hypertension. Garlic has excellent hypotensive qualities. You should consume several cloves (preferably raw) daily. Cayenne pepper is also antihypertensive. Use one teaspoon a day in your cooking if you do not suffer from stomach ulcers. High levels of lead in water have also been linked with hypertension – buy a good water filter.

Supplements which have been found to be useful include:

- *calcium*
- *L-arginine*
- *magnesium*
- *selenium*
- *vitamin C*
- *coenzyme Q10*
- *vitamin E*
- *potassium (not potassium chloride)*
- *garlic capsules – although raw garlic is preferable.*

Include in your diet celery, spinach, onions, oats, rice, wheatgrass, bananas, kumquats, watermelon, shitake mushrooms, flax seeds and chlorella. Oily fish including herring, tuna and salmon are also beneficial so why not try a healthy fish pie with a sweet potato topping.

Stress reduction is vital and deep breathing exercises and regular aromatherapy treatments will help to alleviate anxiety enormously. Regular exercise also helps to reduce states of hypertension.

Only undertake an exercise programme with the permission of your doctor.

The herbs hawthorn berry and mistletoe have a regulating effect on blood pressure but they should be used only under the guidance of a qualified medical herbalist.

Low blood pressure (hypotension)

Hypotension is far less common than hypertension and is regarded as far less serious. However, individuals with chronic hypotension are more prone to dizziness and fainting due to the blood supply to the brain being momentarily interrupted. They may also feel tiredness, fatigue and coldness. Hypotension can be caused by anaemia, hypoglycaemia (low blood sugar), malnutrition or an underactive thyroid.

TREATMENT

Orthodox treatment
Drugs are not usually administered for low blood pressure which is considered not to be dangerous.

Aromatherapy treatment
Essential oils such as **black pepper, hyssop, peppermint, rosemary** and **thyme** may all be used to help to regulate and elevate the blood pressure.

Baths
Daily baths using any of the oils above are excellent for stimulating the circulation and aiding hypotension.

Insight
My favourite aromablend for use in the bath for low blood pressure is two drops black pepper, two drops rosemary and two drops thyme.

Inhalations
Sprinkle two drops rosemary or two drops thyme onto a tissue and inhale several times a day.

Aromamassage
Stimulating massage will help to improve the circulatory system generally. Suggested combinations are:

1 drop black pepper			1 drop hyssop			diluted in
1 drop peppermint	}	or	1 drop rosemary	}		10 ml of
1 drop rosemary			1 drop thyme			carrier oil

Contraindications
Avoid **hyssop** and **thyme** in pregnancy. Do not use **hyssop** excessively in epilepsy. Avoid **peppermint** if taking homoeopathic medication.

BACH FLOWER REMEDIES

Olive is useful for combating fatigue and **Hornbeam** is useful for those 'Monday morning' feelings. Personally, I have found **Scleranthus** to be useful.

DIET

Avoid junk food. A high-protein diet may be beneficial as are leafy green vegetables, soya products, wheatgerm and baked potatoes, which may help to restore elasticity to the arteries and normalize blood pressure.

Supplements of hawthorn berries and mistletoe may be prescribed by a qualified herbalist but should not be taken without supervision.

Siberian ginseng may also normalize blood pressure. Liquorice and nettle tea are also helpful.

Poor circulation

Poor circulation is one of the most common problems that I have come across. I estimate that at least 25 per cent of my clients also suffer from deficient circulation. This condition particularly affects the hands and the feet.

SYMPTOMS

- ▶ *tingling feet*
- ▶ *cramps in hands and/or feet*
- ▶ *leg ulcers*
- ▶ *skin problems*
- ▶ *memory loss.*

TREATMENT

Orthodox treatment
In severe cases drugs may be prescribed to help the circulation. Tests may be carried out to exclude any underlying disease.

Aromatherapy treatment
Essential oils are extremely powerful for stimulating the circulation, causing the capillaries to widen so that a greater volume of blood can flow through them. Particularly effective oils include: **angelica seed, benzoin, black pepper, cardamom, cinnamon, coriander, eucalyptus, geranium, ginger, hyssop, juniper, lemon, mandarin, marjoram, myrtle, niaouli, pine, rosemary** and **thyme.**

Baths
Any of the essential oils suggested above may be added to your bath (six drops). Footbaths and hand baths are also invigorating for the circulation. If you are brave, try plunging your feet alternately into hot and cold footbaths.

> **Insight**
>
> Try the following in a foot or hand bath to improve poor circulation – two drops black pepper, two drops ginger and two drops lemon.

Aromamassage

Daily massage of the hands and the feet improves the circulation dramatically. Clients who have regular aromatherapy treatments often report vast improvements in circulation. Suggested formulae are:

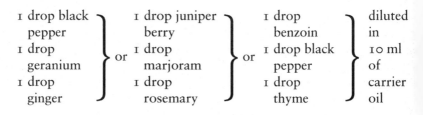

1 drop black pepper
1 drop geranium
1 drop ginger

or

1 drop juniper berry
1 drop marjoram
1 drop rosemary

or

1 drop benzoin
1 drop black pepper
1 drop thyme

diluted in 10 ml of carrier oil

Contraindications

Hyssop, cinnamon and **thyme** should be avoided in pregnancy. Epileptics should avoid excessive use of **hyssop**. Do not use **thyme** excessively in cases of high blood pressure.

BACH FLOWER REMEDIES

Hornbeam and **Olive** may be useful for improving the circulation.

DIET

A healthy diet is essential with plenty of garlic and a teaspoon of cayenne pepper sprinkled on to food daily. Supplements include:

- *gingko biloba which improves the circulation to the head, feet and hands*
- *L-arginine improves circulation by stimulating production of nitric oxide*
- *vitamin C strengthens the capillaries*
- *chromium improves blood circulation*

- *vitamin E*
- *coenzyme Q10*
- *garlic capsules – although raw garlic is preferable*
- *increase intake of bilberries, grapes, basil, dandelion, ginger, rosehip, nettles, rosemary and garlic.*

(You can purchase cordials with extracts of nettle, dandelion, ginger and add them to soups and stews.)

OTHER TREATMENTS

Exercise
Exercise is vital to improve circulation. Rebounding on a mini trampoline is particularly effective, as is skipping, although a brisk walk daily will suffice.

Reflexology
Reflexology is also excellent for improving poor circulation. For those who are unable to exercise it is particularly recommended.

Varicose veins

Varicose veins are dilated, tortuous veins in the legs affecting four times as many women as men. Nearly 50 per cent of middle-aged adults suffer from varicose veins, with the veins just under the skin of the legs most commonly affected. If the deep venous valves or the valves between the deep and superficial valves are incompetent then blood leaks from the deep system to the superficial resulting in varicosity.

Long periods of standing and/or heavy lifting, pregnancy, obesity, damage or genetic weakness of the veins or venous valves, and increased straining and constipation can lead to the development of varicose veins.

If the involved vein is near to the surface, varicose veins are considered not to be harmful, although cosmetically they are unsightly.

If a varicose vein ruptures it will cause severe bleeding. Apply pressure and raise the limb to stop the bleeding – never use a tourniquet.

SYMPTOMS

- *weary, heavy, aching sensation in the lower legs which increases as the day progresses, especially if standing up*
- *pain over the varices*
- *swelling of the ankle and itching skin (due to leakage of the red cells)*
- *pigmentation and ulceration of the skin*
- *leg cramps while lying down.*

TREATMENT

Orthodox treatment
Support stockings are prescribed and injections and various surgical procedures are carried out including 'vein stripping'.

Aromatherapy treatment
The main objective of aromatherapy treatment is to improve the general tone of the veins and to strengthen the circulatory system.

Baths
Cypress (in particular), **geranium** and **lemon** are the three essential oils that I usually select for the treatment of varicose veins. Other alternatives are **black pepper, ginger, juniper, lavender, peppermint, rosemary** and **sandalwood**. Take daily baths using one or a combination of the oils above – it may take many months before any improvement is evident. Suggested formulae include:

2 drops cypress		2 drops ginger
2 drops geranium	or	2 drops juniper berry
2 drops lavender		2 drops rosemary

Aromamassage

Perform aromamassage extremely gently over an area of varicose veins, effleuraging from the ankle to the thigh. Employ massage particularly above the affected area of the vein. You can add essential oils to a pure organic skin cream and apply this daily. Dab the cream gently on to the affected area. The following massage blends should help to prevent as well as to alleviate varicose veins:

1 drop cypress		1 drop cypress		diluted in
1 drop geranium	or	1 drop juniper berry		10 ml of carrier
1 drop lemon		1 drop lavender		oil/lotion

Contraindications

Avoid **lemon** prior to sunbathing.

BACH FLOWER REMEDIES

Olive is useful for the tiredness in the legs. **Impatiens** can help to relieve the pain and **Crab Apple** is the remedy to clear away any feelings of dislike that one may have about the appearance of the varicose veins.

DIET

A high-fibre diet is important for the treatment and prevention of varicose veins. Individuals who have a low-fibre diet, high in refined foods, have a tendency to strain during bowel movements which increases the pressure in the abdomen and obstructs the flow of blood up the legs. This increased pressure weakens the vein wall, leading to the formation of varicose veins and/or haemorrhoids. A high-fibre diet will ensure that the stools are soft and easy to pass without straining.

Include lots of garlic in the diet (especially raw) to improve the circulatory system. Eat plenty of fresh fruit, vegetables, legumes and grains, especially foods such as blackberries, blackcurrants, bilberry, citrus fruits, cherries, pineapples, rosehips, strawberries, raw peppers and green leafy vegetables. The berries will help to reduce the fragility of the capillaries and increase the muscular tone of the veins.

Obviously you should avoid junk food as well as strong tea and coffee.

Supplements include:

- *gingko biloba to improve the circulation*
- *vitamin C strengthens the capillaries*
- *vitamin E*
- *grapeseed extract*
- *garlic capsules – although raw garlic is preferable*
- *horse chestnut*
- *noni juice.*

Try juicing apples and blueberries and make a smoothie including pineapple, bio yoghurt and strawberries as well.

OTHER TREATMENTS

Insight

I always advise my clients who suffer with varicose veins to rest with the legs higher than the head for at least 15 minutes every day to improve drainage and to alleviate the uncomfortable aching sensation. The best position is to lie on the floor with the legs and feet up on a chair.

Exercise

Avoid standing in one place for long periods of time. Walking, cycling and swimming are particularly suitable forms of exercise.

Oils for other circulatory disorders

The following essential oils may be applied, using any of the methods outlined in Chapter 3. Daily baths, footbaths or hand baths in combination with regular aromatherapy massage are particularly recommended.

Arteriosclerosis

Black pepper, ginger, juniper, lemon, rosemary and yarrow.

Blood purifying
Angelica seed, carrot seed, cypress, eucalyptus, fennel, grapefruit, juniper, lemon and rose.

Chilblains
Black pepper, ginger, lemon and marjoram.

Fever
Angelica seed, bergamot, black pepper, German/Roman chamomile, eucalyptus, ginger, juniper, lavender, marjoram and peppermint.

Heart tonic
Angelica seed, benzoin, lavender, marjoram, melissa, rose and sandalwood.

High cholesterol
Cedarwood, geranium, ginger, juniper, lemon, rosemary and thyme.

Immune system booster
Angelica seed, cajeput, German/Roman chamomile, cinnamon, lavender, lemon, lemongrass, lime, mandarin, myrtle, niaouli, petitgrain, ravensara, tea tree and thyme.

Lymphatic congestion
Angelica seed, black pepper, cardamom, cedarwood, German/Roman chamomile, coriander, cypress, fennel, geranium, grapefruit, juniper, lavender, lemon, lime, pine, rosemary and thyme.

Myalgic encephalomyelitis (ME)
Angelica seed, bergamot, German/Roman chamomile, cinnamon, cypress, lavender, lemon, myrtle, pine, ravensara, rosemary, sandalwood, tea tree and thyme.

Palpitations
German/Roman chamomile, clary sage, lavender, mandarin, melissa, neroli, petitgrain, rose, rosemary, thyme and ylang ylang.

TEST YOUR KNOWLEDGE

1 *What is the treatment for iron deficiency anaemia?*

2 *If you were using black pepper on its own for anaemia how many drops would you put in the bath?*

3 *Which Bach Flower Remedy indicated for exhaustion would be useful for anaemia?*

4 *Raw garlic is helpful for heart and blood pressure problems. How can the breath be sweetened after eating garlic?*

5 *If you were making up an aromamassage blend for high blood pressure using an equal number of drops of frankincense and lavender how many drops of each would you blend in 20 ml of carrier oil?*

6 *Which of the following blends could be used on a daily basis in the bath to help low blood pressure?*
   a *3 drops clary sage/3 drops ylang*
   b *3 drops thyme/3 drops rosemary*

7 *For a footbath or hand bath to treat poor circulation how many drops of ginger would you add?*

8 *Which of the following massage blends could improve varicose veins?*
   a *cypress, lemon and geranium*
   b *lavender, neroli and ylang ylang*

10

Digestion

In this chapter you will learn:
- *the causes and effects of some common digestive disorders*
- *the orthodox treatment for these conditions*
- *which essential oils to use for digestive problems*
- *which Bach Flower Remedies to take*
- *how diet and lifestyle can relieve digestive problems.*

Anorexia nervosa (and bulimia)

Anorexia is most common in teenage girls who become obsessed with their weight. Many sufferers are middle class and of above average intelligence. Anorexia is on the increase and is now also affecting boys.

SYMPTOMS

▶ *persistent, active refusal to eat, sometimes accompanied by self-induced vomiting after food and laxative abuse*
▶ *alterations in body image – anorexics often wear loose clothing to hide their painfully thin frames*
▶ *amenorrhoea (loss of menstruation), slow pulse, decreased body temperature, loss of breasts and infertility*
▶ *constipation can become a problem*
▶ *depressive, obsessional thoughts, low self-esteem, inclined towards perfection*
▶ *obsessions with various forms of exercise.*

Bulimia is a syndrome related to anorexia. The bulimic repeatedly binges on food and then induces vomiting. Without treatment anorexia and bulimia can be fatal.

TREATMENT

Orthodox treatment
Referral to a psychiatrist. Drug therapy such as antidepressants and tranquillizers. Admission to a hospital to achieve a target weight and, in severe cases, tube-feeding.

Aromatherapy treatment
When the anorexic can accept that treatment is required, aromatherapy can be highly successful. Psychotherapy or counselling should be used in conjunction with aromatherapy. The main aim of the treatment is to improve the psychological state of the anorexic. You must develop a trusting relationship if you are to make headway.

Baths
The following essential oils will help to alleviate depression, encourage optimism and improve self-esteem: **bergamot, German/ Roman chamomile, clary sage, frankincense, jasmine, lavender, neroli, rose** and **ylang ylang.**

Angelica seed, bergamot, coriander and **fennel** can be used to help regulate the appetite. **Juniper** will help cleanse the mind of the negative irrational thoughts and feelings of worthlessness.

For courage try **black pepper, fennel, juniper, lavender, marjoram, melissa, myrrh, peppermint, rose** and **thyme.**

For boosting energy levels and to combat feelings of being 'run down', **black pepper, peppermint, rosemary** and **thyme** are also favourable.

Constipation can be treated with **black pepper, fennel, ginger, lemon, mandarin, marjoram, rose** and **rosemary.**

....

Insight

An excellent blend for an aromabath to help someone suffering with an easting disorder would be three drops bergamot, two drops juniper and one drop rose.

....

Aromamassage

Perform aromamassage weekly. As the treatment progresses encourage the anorexic to employ some self-massage techniques. This is an excellent therapy and allows the sufferer to get in touch with his or her body and to learn to love and appreciate him or herself. It engenders a feeling of pampering and restores self-esteem and confidence. Suggested formulae:

1 drop bergamot		1 drop angelica seed		diluted in
1 drop jasmine	or	1 drop neroli		10 ml of
1 drop rose		1 drop rose		carrier oil

For constipation the following formula is suggested and should be massaged into the abdomen in a clockwise direction:

1 drop black pepper		diluted in
1 drop fennel		10 ml of
1 drop rose		carrier oil

Contraindications

Avoid **fennel** and **thyme** if pregnant. Epileptics should not use **fennel** excessively. Do not use **thyme** excessively if there is high blood pressure.

BACH FLOWER REMEDIES

These Remedies are valuable for treating the negative states of mind which surround the anorexic. **Gorse** will help to restore hope if the anorexic is totally pessimistic. **Crab Apple** cleanses away feelings of ugliness, self-disgust, self-hatred and obsessions with body shape. It also reduces the hatred of food, and the feeling that food will contaminate the body. **Willow** is useful for those who feel that they are victims and who dwell upon their misfortunes. **Pine** is the remedy for the guilt, and **Mimulus** counteracts the fear of eating. **Larch** is essential for restoring confidence. **Olive** is useful for boosting energy levels.

DIET

To gain weight the anorexic should eat small but frequent meals of nutrient-rich foods. Fruit and vegetables will probably not seem too much of a threat to the anorexic as they are regarded as 'slimming' foods. Nuts and other forms of protein are required to build up the body. Supplements of zinc help to restore the appetite and work on the psychological symptoms. Vitamin B complex, vitamin C, calcium and magnesium are also helpful. Increase zinc-rich foods (lentils, pumpkin seeds, almonds, tofu) and iron-rich foods (beans and pulses, cabbage). Supplements of phosphorus, biotin and B1 may be helpful. Sprouting seeds are fun, easy and nutritious (see pages 188–91).

Candida

Candida albicans, a type of yeast, is present in all of us. Normally the yeast lives harmlessly in the gastrointestinal tract (gut). However, if the yeast multiplies and overgrows it can migrate to the genito-urinary, endocrine, nervous and immune systems. Around a third of the Western world suffers from candida.

SYMPTOMS

- *thrush (of the vagina or mouth), bloating, flatulence, anal itching, altered bowel function (constipation and diarrhoea), heartburn*
- *headaches and migraine*
- *fatigue and lethargy*
- *depression, irritability, poor concentration*
- *allergies and low immune function*
- *PMS and other menstrual irregularities*
- *skin problems – acne, skin rashes, hives.*

The main cause of candida is prolonged antibiotic therapy which destroys the body's 'friendly bacteria' especially in the digestive tract, and promotes the overgrowth of candida. Oral contraceptives and corticosteroids also encourage the proliferation of candida. A person with low immune function is also more susceptible to the disease.

TREATMENT

Orthodox treatment
Antifungal drugs and pessaries will be prescribed.

Aromatherapy treatment
The following essential oils are highly effective for eliminating candida: **German/Roman chamomile, cinnamon, ginger, lavender, myrrh, patchouli, rosemary, tea tree, thyme** and **yarrow.**

Baths
Daily baths or local applications are essential. You may need to continue these for a period of months before the candida is under control. Suggested formulae:

2 drops lavender 2 drops myrrh 2 drops tea tree	or	2 drops German chamomile 2 drops patchouli 2 drops tea tree	or	2 drops lavender 2 drops thyme 2 drops yarrow

The above essential oils may also be used in a sitz bath if the main problem is vaginal thrush.

Insight
For oral thrush I recommend adding two drops of any of the suggested oils to a glass of water and gargling several times a day. Try one drop of myrrh and one drop of tea tree.

Aromamassage
Although the local applications already described are valuable, aromamassage is also recommended. Perform abdominal massage

to balance the constipation and diarrhoea. If constipation is the main problem then **black pepper, ginger, rosemary** and **thyme** may be used. If diarrhoea is present then try **German/Roman chamomile, patchouli** and **yarrow**.

For headaches and migraines **German/Roman chamomile, lavender** and **peppermint** will help to relieve the pain.

Tea tree, lavender, lemon, sandalwood and **yarrow** boost the immune system. The fatigue and lethargy which is so much associated with candida will respond to **cinnamon, ginger, rosemary, tea tree** and **thyme**.

Poor concentration and memory loss will benefit from essential oils of **basil, peppermint** and **rosemary**.

Yoghurt
Yoghurt is wonderfully soothing and cooling and can help to relieve itching. It also regulates the friendly bacteria.

1 drop German chamomile ⎫ added to a
1 drop myrrh   ⎬ carton of 'live'
1 drop tea tree   ⎭ yoghurt

Another form of treatment involves the application of yoghurt mixture to the vaginal area, endeavouring to get it into the vagina. A tampon may be soaked in the yoghurt mixture and inserted into the vagina twice daily to help alleviate symptoms of vaginal thrush.

Contraindications
Avoid **myrrh, cinnamon** and **thyme** during pregnancy. Do not use **thyme** excessively in cases of high blood pressure. Avoid **lemon** prior to sunbathing.

BACH FLOWER REMEDIES

Olive is a remedy for extreme fatigue and lethargy. **Crab Apple** is ideal for cleansing the candida fungus from the system. **Mustard**

is helpful for bouts of depression and **Impatiens** soothes states of anger and irritability.

DIET

The diet should be free from all refined sugar as well as fruit juices and honey, as candida thrives on high sugar levels. Avoid foods containing yeast or made with yeast, as well as any foods containing mould such as mushrooms (shitake mushrooms are candida albicans free) and mouldy cheeses. Antibiotics should also be eliminated as much as possible under medical supervision.

Eat plenty of organic live, low-fat plain yoghurt which will regulate the friendly bacteria, and garlic and ginger, which are antifungal. Cinnamon, rosemary, lemongrass, oregano and thyme also kill bacteria.

Supplements include acidophilus and bifidobacteria to replace the good bacteria and caprylic acid to inhibit yeast overgrowth. Iron and zinc are helpful and propolis and spirulina may also be useful. Activated charcoal (20–30 g daily with a meal) may also be beneficial.

Soups can be very cleansing – try a broth of fresh onion, parsley, thyme, oregano, lemongrass and carrot. Boil for 30 minutes and drink the broth throughout the day.

Constipation

Constipation can be defined as the difficult or infrequent passing of motions. Some of the most common causes of constipation include:

- *poor diet (high in refined foods and low in fibre) and inadequate fluid intake*
- *inadequate exercise or prolonged bed rest*
- *drugs – laxatives or enema (abuse), antibiotics, antacids, steroids, painkillers, antidepressants, diuretics.*

SYMPTOMS

▶ *infrequent bowel movements*
▶ *difficulty passing stools*
▶ *discomfort and pain in the abdomen*
▶ *nausea.*

TREATMENT

Orthodox treatment
The doctor may prescribe laxatives or suppositories and may give advice on diet. Enemas are occasionally necessary.

Aromatherapy treatment
A large number of essential oils are helpful for the relief of constipation. These include: **black pepper, cardamom, cinnamon, fennel, ginger, hyssop, juniper, lemon, marjoram, patchouli, rose, rosemary** and **thyme.**

Baths
Daily baths with any of the oils suggested above will be beneficial.

Aromamassage
Aromamassage of the abdomen is by far the most effective aromatherapy treatment for constipation. Perform this twice daily where the problem is chronic; when the bowel has been retrained it can be performed whenever necessary. Commence at the bottom right-hand side of the abdomen working up the ascending colon using your three middle fingers to gently massage the colon. Use small, circular movements. Proceed across the abdomen to stimulate the transverse colon, and to complete your colon massage work down the descending colon to the left-hand side of the abdomen (you can perform these movements in the bath as well as with a massage blend). You should never experience extreme discomfort.

Some of the best combinations of essential oils are:

1 drop fennel 1 drop marjoram 1 drop rosemary	or	1 drop black pepper 1 drop marjoram 1 drop patchouli	or	1 drop cardamom 1 drop fennel 1 drop juniper berry	diluted in 10 ml of carrier oil

Although constipation may be caused by physical reasons such as poor diet and lack of exercise, bear in mind that it can be caused by emotional problems which have been suppressed. For these individuals, full body aromatherapy treatments are extremely worthwhile to encourage a 'letting-go' of all the emotional baggage and to reduce stress, anxiety and shock. The following combinations work on a physical, emotional and spiritual level:

1 drop juniper berry 1 drop marjoram 1 drop rose	or	1 drop bergamot 1 drop frankincense 1 drop rose	diluted in 10 ml of carrier oil

Contraindications

Do not use **cinnamon, fennel, hyssop, marjoram** or **thyme** excessively in pregnancy. **Fennel** and **hyssop** should be avoided by epileptics. Avoid **bergamot** prior to sunbathing. Do not use **thyme** excessively in cases of high blood pressure.

BACH FLOWER REMEDIES

The Bach Flower Remedy **Crab Apple** is valuable for cleansing and for anyone who feels disgust at bodily functions, dislikes themselves or considers themselves to be dirty or ugly. **Mimulus** can be used to help counteract the fear that passing a motion will be painful or that blood may be passed. **Agrimony** should be taken if an individual feels tortured and tormented inside. **Pine** is for the release of guilt and **Honeysuckle** is for letting go of the past. **Walnut** stimulates change and, therefore, helps to retrain the bowel.

Dietary changes are vital and you should eat a healthy, high-fibre diet to retrain the bowel. Dietary fibre increases both the frequency and quantity of bowel movements. Consume plenty of fruit and vegetables, as well as pulses, cereals, nuts and seeds – this is vital! Drink six to eight glasses of water daily. Never repress an urge to defecate, and you should never strain. You can use laxative herbs to re-establish bowel activity but do not abuse them. Cascara, cassia, senna, psyllium seed husks and aloe vera have long been used as laxatives. You can drink several cups of fennel and ginger tea daily to stimulate the bowel, and green tea is also beneficial.

Insight

Lactobacillus acidophilus benefits 90 per cent of constipation sufferers and lignans (from flax seeds), chitocan, cellulose, psyllium help to relieve symptoms too.

Iron, calcium and vitamin C intake should be increased and beneficial fruits are apricots, bananas, figs, grapefruit, lemon, prunes and watermelon. Avocado, beetroot, cabbage, carrot, spinach and turnip are useful too.

Soups and smoothies are a great way to incorporate a large number of these foods. Regular exercise can also help to alleviate constipation. A brisk walk every day is ideal.

Heartburn/acid stomach/indigestion (dyspepsia)

The above conditions can be induced by a variety of factors:

▶ *overindulgence in food and/or drink, rushing or not chewing food*
▶ *too much stress and tension which increases stomach acid*
▶ *an underlying disease – seek medical advice if symptoms persist.*

SYMPTOMS

▶ *a burning sensation or discomfort behind the breastbone which may spread up the oesophagus to the back of the mouth.*

TREATMENT

Orthodox treatment
Antacids will be prescribed and if symptoms persist, you may be referred to hospital for a barium meal.

Aromatherapy treatment
Dietary changes will be necessary but essential oils can provide relief from acidity and indigestion. Invaluable essential oils are: **angelica seed, basil, bergamot, black pepper, cardamom, carrot seed, German/Roman chamomile, cinnamon, coriander, fennel, juniper, lavender, lemon, marjoram, peppermint** and **rosemary.**

Baths
Take daily baths using three drops lemon and three drops ginger or three drops lemon and three drops peppermint, depending on your aroma preference.

Compresses
A warm compress using one or a combination of the oils above can be comforting if placed over the stomach.

2 drops German/Roman chamomile		
2 drops fennel	or	2 drops cardamom
2 drops lemon		2 drops ginger
		2 drops spearmint

Insight

To combat heartburn you may also make up teas of dill, fennel, lemon or peppermint. Place one drop of any of these essential oils into a glass of warm water to which you have added a teaspoon of honey. Another idea is to squeeze half a lemon into a glass of water.

Aromamassage

To alleviate the discomfort and pain, you may apply a blend of essential oils to the abdominal area, under the ribcage and around the throat area.

1 drop carrot seed	}	or	2 drops fennel	}	diluted in 10
1 drop lemon			1 drop		ml of carrier
1 drop ginger			peppermint		oil

If the indigestion is being caused by anxiety and worry, a different combination of essential oils is required:

1 drop German/Roman	}	or	2 drops	}	diluted in
chamomile			bergamot		10 ml of
1 drop marjoram			1 drop rose		carrier oil
1 drop neroli					

Contraindications

Avoid **fennel** and **marjoram** if epileptic. Avoid **bergamot** prior to sunbathing. Avoid **fennel** and **cinnamon** if pregnant.

BACH FLOWER REMEDIES

Rescue Remedy can be taken to reduce stress and tension if this is the cause.

DIET

Eat slowly, chew thoroughly and try not to overeat too many heavy, rich meals. Try not to eat too many acid-forming foods which include biscuits, bread, cake, dairy foods, meat, pasta, sugar, alcohol, coffee and tea. Eat more alkaline-forming foods such as fresh fruit, vegetables and salad. Experiment with proper 'food combining', not mixing carbohydrate and protein together in the same meal.

Slippery elm and bentonite clay have been proven to be useful, and juicing cabbage and potato is beneficial – do a ten-day course of this to see the benefits. Try to ensure that meal times are not stressful and not too late at night.

Obesity

Obesity is defined as a condition in which an individual's weight is 20 per cent or more above the ideal weight. It is a major problem in our society and affects approximately one-third of adults in Britain.

SYMPTOMS

This condition carries with it many adverse effects on health including reduced life expectancy, increased blood pressure, elevated cholesterol, risk of heart disease, late onset diabetes, digestive problems, arthritis and problems with the weight-bearing joints such as the knees or the hips. The obese individual also experiences much psychological trauma such as low self-esteem, depression, overeating for consolation and social rejection.

Although occasionally obesity is caused by disorders such as underactive thyroid, the majority of individuals are obese because they eat more than they need to maintain their normal level of activity.

TREATMENT

Orthodox treatment
A slimming diet should be followed in conjunction with an exercise programme. In several cases of obesity radical surgery may be performed to reduce calorie intake, such as stapling the stomach. Such procedures are only used if the person's life is in danger.

Aromatherapy treatment
We all over-indulge sometimes – Christmas is a prime example – and so essential oils that help us to lose weight are welcome. These include: **black pepper, cardamom, cypress, fennel, geranium, ginger, grapefruit, juniper, lemon, patchouli, peppermint** and **rosemary.**

Insight

Fennel is probably the most useful oil for aiding weight loss and it has had a reputation of suppressing hunger since Roman and Greek times. Men ate fennel to give them energy and to allay hunger while on marches. Women ate fennel to prevent weight gain. Throughout the Middle Ages fennel was a permitted herb on fasting days. Fennel is a detoxifying oil and also an excellent diuretic and so helps to rid the body of any excessive fluids.

Black pepper and **rosemary** are powerful stimulants and tonics and, therefore, help to give the metabolism a 'kick start'. **Juniper** is a remarkable detoxifier and is also a diuretic. **Cypress, grapefruit** and **lemon** also help to cleanse the body and reduce excess fluid. **Cardamom** and **peppermint** help the digestion.

After weight loss has been achieved the skin can become loose and saggy. Essential oils such as **black pepper, frankincense, lavender, lemongrass, mandarin, myrrh, patchouli** and **rosemary** may help.

Always consider the psychological state of the obese individual. Uplifting oils to improve self-esteem and to build up confidence and positivity are vital. The 'luxurious' oils such as **jasmine, rose** and **neroli** are particularly valuable. But if funds are low then **bergamot, German/Roman chamomile, geranium, lavender** and **mandarin** are all beneficial.

Unfortunately essential oils will not miraculously dissolve away fat! They must, of course, be used in combination with a sensible diet.

Baths
Aromatherapy baths should be preceded by dry skin brushing. This will help to speed up the process of elimination and will unclog the pores of the skin and the lymphatic system. It will also improve the circulation. It should be performed at least once a day, brushing from the periphery of the body towards the centre and the heart.

Suggested blends for the baths to encourage detoxification and to dispel fluid retention are:

2 drops cypress 2 drops fennel 2 drops rosemary	} or	2 drops black pepper 2 drops geranium 2 drops lemon	} or	2 drops ginger 2 drops juniper berry 2 drops peppermint	

To uplift anxiety and depression:

2 drops bergamot
2 drops geranium   }
2 drops rose

Aromamassage

The use of aromamassage will help to change the way overweight people feel about themselves, encouraging a positive body image. Regular massage will also help to improve the appearance of the skin and stimulate muscle tone. A weekly full body massage is recommended, paying particular attention to the 'problem' areas. Some blends which you can experiment with are:

2 drops bergamot 1 drop fennel 1 drop rose 2 drops geranium 1 drop juniper berry	diluted in 20 ml of carrier oil	or	1 drop cypress 1 drop ginger 2 drops mandarin 1 drop peppermint	diluted in 15 ml of carrier oil

Contraindications

Avoid **fennel** in pregnancy and in cases of epilepsy. Do not apply **bergamot** or **grapefruit** prior to sunbathing.

BACH FLOWER REMEDIES

Crab Apple is the remedy to improve self-image, cleansing away any thoughts of self-disgust and ugliness. **Larch** is indicated for lack of confidence. **Impatiens** is the remedy to help if there is impatience with slow weight loss. **Chestnut Bud** is for those individuals who have tried to diet many times before yet have reverted to their old ways. **Chestnut Bud** helps you learn from your past experiences. **Gorse** helps to engender hope and positivity.

DIET

A diet low in fibre, high in refined carbohydrates and fats is the main reason for obesity in the West. Avoid saturated fats such as butter, lard and animal fats. Stop snacking on high-sugar foods such as biscuits, cakes and sweets. The diet should be high in fibre which tends to be filling, not fattening, and full of nutrients. Fruit, vegetables, salads, pulses and wholegrains are highly recommended. Drink dandelion, fennel or ginger tea and green tea to help weight loss. Pay attention to portion control and plan ahead with a meal planner when shopping. Do not be tempted by the crisp and cookie aisle!

Add spirulina and diakon into your plan. Diakon helps dissolve hard fat deposits from the tissues and coconut oil is also beneficial. Try a cleansing broth; juicing and sprouting are helpful too. It is important to combine a healthy diet with an exercise programme for optimum results. A brisk walk daily will suffice, although swimming and cycling are also appropriate activities.

Try to be patient! If the weight loss is achieved gradually it is more likely to be permanent. If there is little or no decrease in weight during the first month, however, check with your doctor that you do not have a thyroid condition or another problem that makes weight reduction difficult.

Oils for other digestive disorders

The following essential oils may be applied, using any of the methods outlined in Chapter 3. Gentle massage of the abdomen and compresses are particularly effective for digestive disorders.

Colic

Basil, benzoin, bergamot, black pepper, cardamom, German/Roman chamomile, cinnamon, clary sage, coriander, fennel, frankincense, ginger, juniper, lavender, lemon, lemongrass, mandarin, marjoram, melissa, myrrh, peppermint, rosemary and yarrow.

Colitis

Bergamot, black pepper, cardamom, cinnamon, cajeput, German/Roman chamomile, coriander, fennel, juniper, lavender, lemongrass, neroli, peppermint, rosemary, tea tree and yarrow.

Diabetes

Eucalyptus, geranium and juniper.

Diarrhoea

Black pepper, cajeput, German/Roman chamomile, cinnamon, coriander, cypress, eucalyptus, geranium, ginger, juniper, lavender, lemon, mandarin, myrrh, myrtle, neroli, niaouli, patchouli, peppermint, rosemary and sandalwood.

Fistula (anal)

Geranium, lavender, lemon and tea tree.

Flatulence

Angelica seed, basil, bergamot, cardamom, carrot seed, cinnamon, German/Roman chamomile, coriander, fennel, ginger, hyssop, lemon, marjoram, neroli, peppermint, rosemary and thyme.

Food poisoning

Black pepper, fennel, grapefruit, juniper, lemon and peppermint.

Gall bladder

Bergamot, carrot seed, German/Roman chamomile, geranium, lavender, lemon, peppermint, rose, rosemary, yarrow and ylang ylang.

Gastritis

German/Roman chamomile, lavender, lemon, melissa, sandalwood and yarrow.

Gastro-enteritis
Basil, bergamot, cajeput, German/Roman chamomile, fennel, geranium, lavender, peppermint, rosemary, tea tree, thyme and yarrow.

Halitosis (bad breath)
Bergamot, coriander, fennel, lemon, parsley seed, peppermint and spearmint.

Hangover
Fennel, ginger, juniper and rosemary.

Hiccoughs
Basil, fennel and mandarin.

Liver
Carrot seed, German/Roman chamomile, cypress, geranium, grapefruit, lavender, lemon, mandarin, melissa, peppermint, rose, rosemary, thyme and yarrow.

Loss of appetite
Angelica seed, basil, bergamot, black pepper, caraway, cardamom, German/Roman chamomile, cinnamon, coriander, fennel, ginger, hyssop, juniper, lemon, myrrh, peppermint and thyme.

Nausea/vomiting
Basil, black pepper, cardamom, German/Roman chamomile, cinnamon, coriander, fennel, ginger, lavender, mandarin, melissa and peppermint.

Sluggish digestion
Black pepper, cardamom, cinnamon, coriander, fennel, ginger, grapefruit, juniper and peppermint.

Spleen
Black pepper, German/Roman chamomile, rosemary and thyme.

Stomach ulcers
German/Roman chamomile, geranium, lavender, lemon, peppermint, rosemary and spearmint.

Travel sickness
Ginger, lavender, mandarin, peppermint and spearmint.

Worms and intestinal parasites
Bergamot, cajeput, cardamom, coriander, eucalyptus, fennel, geranium, juniper, lavender, melissa, myrrh, peppermint, rosemary, tea tree and thyme.

TEST YOUR KNOWLEDGE

1   Is aromatherapy particularly useful for the physiological or the psychological state of an anorexic?

2   Which of the following blends is useful for alleviating depression and improving self-esteem in cases of anorexia?
    a   jasmine/rose
    b   niaouli/ravensara

3   Would you use peppermint/fennel or myrrh/tea tree for vaginal thrush?

4   What needs to be eliminated from the diet if a person is suffering from candida?

5   For constipation, which blend would be most beneficial for an aromamassage of the abdomen?
    a   fennel/juniper/marjoram
    b   angelica seed/chamomile/lavender

6   How would you use a lemon for indigestion?

7   Which oil is probably most useful for aiding weight loss, suppressing the appetite and detoxification?

8   Which Bach Flower Remedy is indicated for cleansing and improving self-image in cases of obesity?

11

Muscles and joints

In this chapter you will learn:
- *the causes and effects of the most common muscular and joint problems*
- *the orthodox treatment for these disorders*
- *how aromatherapy may help and why*
- *which Bach Flower Remedies to take*
- *how diet and lifestyle changes can help.*

Arthritis – osteoarthritis

Osteoarthritis is a common degenerative disorder of the joints which occurs in almost everyone over the age of 60. The average age of onset is 50 years. The principal joints which are affected are the weight-bearing joints (i.e. knees and hips) and the joints of the hands. The cartilage is destroyed, exposing the underlying bone, and bony spurs called osteophytes are formed. It is the result of 'wear and tear'.

SYMPTOMS

The main features are stiffness (especially in the morning), pain on moving the involved joint, limitation of movement and deformity.

TREATMENT

Orthodox treatment
Simple analgesics and non-steroidal anti-inflammatory drugs (NSAIDS) are prescribed. As these drugs are associated with

side-effects such as gastrointestinal upset, headaches and dizziness they should be used only for short periods of time. Joint replacement surgery is offered where there is serious degeneration.

Aromatherapy treatment
Aromatherapy is a highly effective treatment for this condition. It can reduce the pain of arthritis and also can improve and maintain the mobility of the joints.

Once again, aromatherapy must be used in conjunction with dietary changes. Start treatment as soon as possible in the early stages of the disease to achieve maximum effect.

Essential oils for arthritis include:

- *Analgesic (pain killing) oils:* **angelica seed, benzoin, cajeput, cardamom, German/Roman chamomile, eucalyptus, frankincense, geranium, ginger, lavender, marjoram, niaouli, peppermint, pine** *and* **rosemary.**
- *Detoxifying oils:* **black pepper, cypress, fennel, ginger, grapefruit, hyssop, juniper, lemon, rosemary** *and* **thyme.**
- *Oils to improve the circulation:* **benzoin, black pepper, cardamom, cinnamon, coriander, eucalyptus, geranium, ginger, hyssop, lemon, mandarin, marjoram, niaouli, pine, rosemary** *and* **thyme.**

Baths
Aromatherapy oils should be added to your daily bath. Choose from the lists above or alternate the following arthritic bath formulae:

Warming and analgesic	**Detoxifying**
1 drop benzoin	2 drops cypress
2 drops black pepper	1 drop fennel
1 drop ginger	2 drops juniper berry
2 drops marjoram	1 drop lemon

If the arthritis sufferer has difficulty in getting into the bath then the same formulae may be added to a footbath or a hand bath.

Compresses

These are excellent for providing pain relief. If the pain is acute then use a cold compress. For chronic pain use a hot compress or a combination of hot and cold. To make a compress mix six drops of essential oil into a small bowl of water. Soak a flannel or any piece of absorbent material into the solution. Gently squeeze the compress and apply it to the painful area.

Insight

For easing the discomfort of osteoarthritis I recommend a compress of two drops black pepper, one drop ginger, two drops marjoram and one drop juniper.

Aromamassage

A full treatment will encourage the elimination of the accumulated toxins and improve the circulation with concentration on the particularly painful areas. The arthritis sufferer should gently massage the affected joints every day.

1 drop black pepper
2 drops frankincense
1 drop ginger
2 drops marjoram

or

1 drop eucalyptus
2 drops juniper berry
2 drops lavender
1 drop rosemary

diluted in 20 ml of carrier oil

Contraindications

Do not use **fennel** and **hyssop** excessively in cases of epilepsy. Avoid **lemon** prior to sunbathing. **Thyme** may raise the blood pressure. Avoid **cinnamon** in pregnancy.

BACH FLOWER REMEDIES

Use **Rescue Remedy** for pain relief.

It is vital that individuals with osteoarthritis are not overweight which puts stress and strain on the weight-bearing joints. Avoid refined carbohydrates and keep fats to a minimum. High-fibre foods are recommended. Plants in the deadly nightshade family can affect some arthritics (aubergines, tomatoes, peppers, potatoes and tobacco), so you could cut them out of your diet for a couple of months to see if there is any improvement.

Supplements that may help arthritis are the B vitamins: folic acid and B_{12} to help grip strength, B_5 for joint pain and B_6 to reduce size and inflammation of nodules. Beansprouts, green leafy vegetables, avocados and nuts all contain high levels of B vitamins. Selenium ACE can also alleviate symptoms. Gentle exercise such as yoga is helpful for keeping the joints mobile.

Arthritis – rheumatoid (RA)

This is a chronic inflammatory condition that can affect the entire body although the joints most often involved are the hands, feet, wrists and ankles. Approximately one per cent of males and three per cent of females are affected in the UK and the average age of onset is 35–55.

Insight

What triggers rheumatoid arthritis, an auto-immune reaction, where antibodies develop against components of joint tissues, remains unknown. Genetic susceptibility, lifestyle, diet and food allergies have all been suggested.

SYMPTOMS

The onset is usually gradual, beginning with mild fevers and vague joint pain. Joint symptoms often begin in the hands or feet in a symmetrical way. The involved joints are swollen, painful and stiff. Eventually joints become quite deformed.

TREATMENT

Orthodox treatment
Involves non-steroidal anti-inflammatory drugs (NSAIDS). As these drugs are associated with side-effects such as gastrointestinal upset, headaches and dizziness, they should be used for short periods of time. Joint replacement surgery is offered where there is serious degeneration.

Aromatherapy treatment
Aromatherapy treatment can be successful, particularly if used in combination with dietary therapy, since RA is not found in societies with a 'primitive' diet but is prevalent in those individuals consuming the Western diet.

Treatment should be directed towards reducing the inflammation as well as cleansing and detoxifying the whole body and alleviating pain.

Essential oils for rheumatoid arthritis include:

- *Anti-inflammatory oils:* **German/Roman chamomile, lavender, myrrh, patchouli, peppermint, sandalwood** *and* **yarrow.**
- *Cleansing oils:* **angelica seed, black pepper, cypress, fennel, ginger, hyssop, juniper, lemon, marjoram, pine, rosemary** *and* **thyme.**
- *Pain-relieving oils:* **cajeput, German/Roman chamomile, cardamom, eucalyptus, frankincense, ginger, lavender, marjoram, niaouli, peppermint** *and* **rosemary.**

Baths
Footbaths and hand baths are valuable for RA since this condition most often involves the hands and feet. Concentrate on using the anti-inflammatory oils during the 'flare-ups'. RA footbath/hand bath formulae (for inflammation):

3 drops German/Roman chamomile			2 drops German/Roman chamomile	
1 drop niaouli	}	or	2 drops lavender	}
2 drops yarrow			2 drops peppermint	

The above formulae may of course be used in baths.

Compresses
These are highly effective when placed on inflamed joints. Put three drops of **German/Roman chamomile** and three drops of **lavender/ yarrow** into a small bowl of water. Soak a piece of absorbent material such as a flannel into this solution. Squeeze it out and place it on to the swollen joint(s).

Aromamassage
A full treatment can be beneficial. However, perform only gentle stroking near any inflamed joints – just enough pressure to apply the oil. You can use aromatherapy treatments together – for instance, you can place compresses on the affected joints while other parts of the body are massaged. The following combinations may be useful:

ANTI-INFLAMMATORY MASSAGE FORMULA

2 drops German/Roman chamomile ⎱
2 drops patchouli   ⎰ diluted in 20 ml of carrier oil
2 drops yarrow

CLEANSING MASSAGE FORMULA

1 drop angelica seed   ⎱
1 drop black pepper   ⎰ diluted in 20 ml of carrier oil
1 drop cypress
2 drops juniper berry
1 drop lemon

ANALGESIC MASSAGE FORMULA

1 drop frankincense   ⎱
2 drops ginger   ⎰ diluted in 20 ml of carrier oil
1 drop lavender
1 drop peppermint
1 drop rosemary

Contraindications

Thyme may raise the blood pressure. Do not use **fennel** or **hyssop** excessively in cases of epilepsy. Do not apply **lemon** prior to sunbathing. Avoid **peppermint** when taking homoeopathic medications. Do not use **cinnamon, hyssop** and **fennel** in pregnancy.

BACH FLOWER REMEDIES

Rescue Remedy is useful for pain relief. **Agrimony** is for sufferers of RA who hide their pain behind a happy, brave face.

DIET

Since RA is found in societies consuming a Western diet, nutrition is an important factor. Food allergies can often be implicated in RA. It is well worth avoiding the possible culprits for a while. The most common foods are the nightshade family (tomatoes, peppers, aubergines and potatoes), dairy products and wheat.

The diet should be low in sugar, salt, refined carbohydrates and saturated fats. Eat lots of green vegetables, fruit and oily fish such as mackerel, salmon and sardines. If you have a juicer, carrot, celery, cabbage and alfalfa juices are beneficial. Foods high in selenium (brazil nuts, muesli) are useful as well as foods rich in zinc (lentils, pumpkin seeds). Vitamins A, B, E, K (vitamin K – celery, garlic, lettuce, rhubarb, turnip) may also help. Ground flax seeds, fish oils, borage oil and evening primrose oil all help to alleviate symptoms.

Some RA sufferers benefit from fasting for a few days. Detoxifying oils should be used for this period.

Gout

Gout is caused by an increased level of uric acid, crystals of which are deposited in the joints. It is most common in men over the age of 30 and tends to run in families. Eating too much rich food and drinking too much alcohol may precipitate an attack. Trauma and some drugs may also cause it.

SYMPTOMS

Gout is intensely painful and commonly affects the big toe which will be red, hot, shiny and incredibly painful. Subsequent attacks are fairly common.

TREATMENT

Orthodox treatment
Consists of the administration of anti-inflammatory drugs.

Aromatherapy treatment
This will involve using essential oils to combat the inflammation during the attack. Treatment will be aimed at preventing further attacks of gout and will involve detoxification and changes in diet. Individuals with gout are often obese and they will be encouraged to lose weight to avoid high blood pressure, heart disease and diabetes.

Essential oils for gout include: **angelica seed, basil, cajeput, carrot seed, chamomile, hyssop, juniper, lemon, niaouli, pine, rosemary, thyme** and **yarrow**.

Baths
During an attack the affected joint should never be massaged. Footbaths are, therefore, particularly indicated and they can provide a great deal of pain relief.

Gout footbath formulae:

2 drops angelica seed
2 drops carrot seed   } or
2 drops hyssop

1 drop cajeput
2 drops juniper berry
1 drop lemon
2 drops rosemary

Compresses

Any of the recommended oils above can also be used to make a compress. Put the oils into a bowl of cold water, soak up with a flannel and place on the affected joint.

Insight

My favourite aromacompress for gout is two drops juniper, two drops lemon and two drops yarrow.

Aromamassage

The purpose of the aromamassage is to detoxify and thus maintain uric acid levels within the normal range. Any of the detoxification oils recommended for arthritis may be used. Two drops of each of juniper, lemon, rosemary and thyme is a good combination. If the sufferer is obese, refer to page 229 in this book for recommendations. It would, of course, be contraindicated to massage an area of inflammation such as the big toe.

Contraindications

Thyme can raise the blood pressure. Avoid **lemon** prior to sunbathing. Avoid **hyssop** in pregnancy.

DIET

Attention to diet is essential if gout is to be prevented. Avoid organ meats, red meat and alcohol in particular. Do not eat too much of the following: fats, refined foods, shellfish, yeast, cheese, salt, anchovies, coffee, tea and all foods and drinks containing sugar and fructose. If you are obese, it is vital to lose weight.

Drink plenty of water (two litres daily). Fresh fruit and vegetables are also beneficial.

Cherries and cherry juice alleviate gout by lowering uric acid levels (250 g daily) and fennel, rosemary, rye sprouts, beetroot, celery and lettuce and raw potato juice all help.

Supplements which may be helpful include celery seed extract capsules and vitamin C.

Oils for other muscular/joint disorders

The following essential oils may be applied, using any of the methods outlined in Chapter 3. Gentle massage of the affected area(s), in combination with daily aromatherapy baths, is recommended. Compresses are excellent for pain relief.

Aches and pains
Angelica seed, basil, benzoin, black pepper, cajeput, cardamom, German/Roman chamomile, cinnamon, coriander, eucalyptus, frankincense, geranium, ginger, juniper, lavender, lemon, lemongrass, marjoram, niaouli, peppermint, pine, ravensara, rosemary, thyme, vetivert and yarrow.

Bruises
Black pepper, German/Roman chamomile, fennel, geranium, ginger, hyssop, lavender, marjoram, myrrh, peppermint and rosemary.

Cramp
Basil, black pepper, cajeput, cardamom, German/Roman chamomile, cypress, lavender, marjoram, rosemary and vetivert.

Lack of tone
Black pepper, juniper, lavender, lemongrass and rosemary.

Rheumatism
Angelica seed, basil, benzoin, black pepper, cajeput, caraway, cedarwood, German/Roman chamomile, cinnamon, coriander, cypress, eucalyptus, frankincense, ginger, grapefruit, hyssop, juniper, lavender, lemon, lime, marjoram, myrrh, niaouli, peppermint, pine, rosemary, thyme, vetivert and yarrow.

Sprains and strains
Black pepper, cajeput, German/Roman chamomile, eucalyptus, ginger, hyssop, lavender, lemongrass, marjoram, pine, ravensara, rosemary, thyme, vetivert and yarrow.

TEST YOUR KNOWLEDGE

1 *Which of the following oils would be suitable as analgesia (pain relief) in cases of osteoarthritis?*
   a *black pepper/ginger*
   b *lemon/grapefruit*

2 *Would cypress/fennel or frankincense/lavender be beneficial to encourage the detoxification process and thus improve osteoarthritis?*

3 *To curb inflammation associated with rheumatoid arthritis would you choose chamomile/yarrow or cajeput/rosemary?*

4 *Which joint is most commonly affected by gout?*

5 *Would you massage an inflamed joint?*

12

Skin and hair

In this chapter you will learn:
- *about the main causes of skin and hair problems*
- *how to care for your skin and hair using essential oils*
- *how to create individual aromatherapy blends for your hair and skin type*
- *simple dietary and lifestyle changes to promote healthy skin and hair.*

Commercially produced cosmetics contain synthetic substances such as preservatives, dyes and fragrances which are damaging to the skin's flora and protective 'acid mantle'. They promote ageing of the skin which results in wrinkles.

Commercial shampoos clean so thoroughly that the scalp's natural sebum is washed away. Because the scalp is thrown out of balance the hair is unable to grow as well as it should do. Shampoos also contain preservatives, chemicals, dyes and fragrances which can penetrate the hair follicles and enter the bloodstream. Ready-made cosmetics and shampoos also cost a great deal, far more than home-made natural cosmetics. Advertising and packaging are expensive and the manufacturer and the retailer also have to make a profit, of course.

Cosmetics made with essential oils can promote and protect your natural beauty and have the advantage that you know exactly what is in them.

Insight

It is very satisfying and enjoyable to create your own aromatherapy products, and they do make wonderful gifts for your family and friends. A luxurious facial oil of three drops frankincense, three drops neroli and three drops rose in 30 ml jojoba oil will be greatly appreciated as a Christmas gift!

Skin

WHAT CAUSES SKIN DISORDERS?

Skin problems can be caused by a variety of physical and emotional factors:

- ▶ *poor diet*
- ▶ *deficiency of oxygen from closed, overheated rooms*
- ▶ *environmental pollutants*
- ▶ *chemical pollutants*
- ▶ *food intolerances (e.g. dairy foods, wheat)*
- ▶ *hormone imbalances*
- ▶ *smoking*
- ▶ *drugs*
- ▶ *synthetic cosmetics*
- ▶ *stress and emotional problems*
- ▶ *work or exercise outside in the sun, wind and rain.*

Insight

When tackling skin problems the only real long-term solution is to try to discover the root cause of the disorder rather than just working on the symptoms. A change in living and eating habits is often necessary alongside your essential oil regime. Our skin is a mirror of our inner health.

DRY SKIN CARE

Dry skin is lacking in moisture as the sebaceous glands are inactive and not producing enough sebum. Dry skin, unfortunately, is prone to more wrinkles than any other skin type. It needs to be 'fed' daily with nourishing and protective oils. Vegetable oils with essential oils are the best way to prevent the loss of moisture and to activate the sebaceous glands.

Dry skin base oils: **sweet almond, avocado, evening primrose, jojoba, apricot kernel** and **peach kernel** oils are all excellent skin oil bases. Remember to add a small amount of **wheatgerm oil** to preserve your facial oil.

Essential oils for dry skin: **benzoin, carrot seed, German/Roman chamomile, frankincense, geranium, jasmine, lavender, neroli, palmarosa, rose, rosewood, sandalwood, vetivert, ylang ylang.**

Suggested recipes for dry skin facial oils
You may select any of the essential oils from the list above and add them to your chosen carrier oil(s) or moisturizing lotion. However, you may find the following recipes useful:

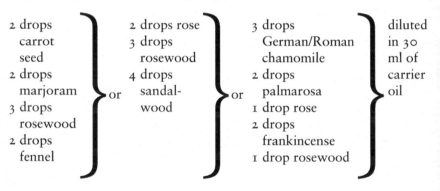

2 drops carrot seed
2 drops marjoram
3 drops rosewood
2 drops fennel

or

2 drops rose
3 drops rosewood
4 drops sandal-wood

or

3 drops German/Roman chamomile
2 drops palmarosa
1 drop rose
2 drops frankincense
1 drop rosewood

diluted in 30 ml of carrier oil

Put all your ingredients into an amber-coloured bottle and shake well prior to use.

Insight
If you have dry skin never use soap and water to cleanse your skin: this will cause further loss of moisture. Your facial oil will make a suitable cleanser. Also avoid hot facial steambaths and hot facial masks.

Lukewarm compresses for dry skin

Lukewarm compresses may be used to cleanse dry skin.

Heat up about a pint of water. Add four drops of essential oil and stir. Dip a face flannel into the solution and place it on your face until the compress cools off. The following recipes are recommended:

2 drops German/Roman
   chamomile
1 drop neroli   } or
1 drop rose

2 drops carrot seed
1 drop rose
1 drop sandalwood   }

This skin type should also avoid all cosmetics containing alcohol which will strip even more moisture from the surface of the skin.

Diet

Eat plenty of fresh fruit and vegetables as well as lots of oily fish. Vitamin C, evening primrose oil and zinc may also help. Increase potassium, zinc, biotin, vitamin A and vitamin E rich foods. Royal Jelly, grapes, chamomile, flax seed oil, avocado, carrots and cucumber will all help liven up dry skin.

Try to avoid dry atmospheres and strong sunlight, wind and sun beds. Do not smoke and drink excessively. Coconut oil applied topically and taken internally is beneficial. Try drinking juices made of grape, cucumber, apple and carrot. It is important to try to avoid stress.

OILY SKIN CARE

Oily skin occurs when the sebaceous glands produce too much sebum. The pores of the skin are often clogged and therefore have a tendency to form spots, blackheads and even acne. Areas particularly affected include the nose, chin and forehead. Oily skin is most common during puberty due to the hormonal changes which are occurring.

Facial steambaths and compresses are highly effective for oily skin. A facial steambath will cleanse the pores thoroughly, flushing out the toxic substances and stimulating the circulation. It should be carried out once a week.

Facial steambath for oily skin
Boil about a litre of water and pour into a bowl. Add approximately six drops of essential oil. Bend your head over the bowl and cover your head with a towel. Steam your face for approximately ten minutes. Suggested recipes:

2 drops cypress   2 drops rosemary   in a bowl of
2 drops lemon   or   2 drops geranium   water
2 drops juniper berry   2 drops tea tree

Face masks are also beneficial for oily skin. They cleanse, tauten and invigorate the skin. The most important ingredient of a face pack is fuller's earth or clay which will pull the toxins out of the skin.

Face mask for oily skin

2 tablespoons of clay/fuller's earth
1 teaspoon lemon pulp
1 teaspoon water
1 teaspoon honey
1 drop cypress
1 drop juniper berry

Mix the above ingredients together to form a paste. Apply to the face avoiding the area around the eyes. Leave the mask on until completely dry. Carefully wash it off using a warm, damp flannel. Give yourself a face mask once a week. Oily skin should also be treated with a vegetable facial oil.

Oily skin base oils: suitable carrier oils include **sweet almond, apricot kernel, peach kernel, evening primrose, borage seed** and **carrot oil.**

Essential oils for oily skin: **bergamot, cedarwood, cypress, frankincense, geranium, juniper, lavender, lemon, palmarosa, petitgrain, rosemary, ylang ylang.**

Suggested recipes for oily skin facial oils
Select any of the essential oils from the list above and add them to your chosen carrier oil(s). However, the following recipes are useful:

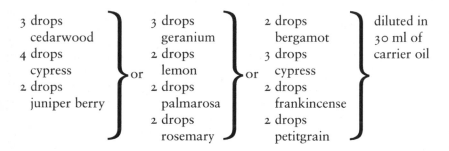

| 3 drops cedarwood 4 drops cypress 2 drops juniper berry | or | 3 drops geranium 2 drops lemon 2 drops palmarosa 2 drops rosemary | or | 2 drops bergamot 3 drops cypress 2 drops frankincense 2 drops petitgrain | diluted in 30 ml of carrier oil |

Put all your ingredients into an amber-coloured bottle and shake well.

Insight

Spots and blackheads may be treated individually with one drop of neat lavender or tea tree. Apply one drop on a cotton bud to the affected area several times a day.

Diet

Oily skin is made worse by a diet rich in fatty foods and sugar. Eat lots of fruit and vegetables and plenty of fibre to avoid constipation which always makes oily skin worse. Drink approximately two litres water daily. Avoid tea, coffee and cigarettes. Aniseed tea internally can be very soothing and raw potato applied topically reduces oiliness. Horseradish juice diluted 50 per cent cleanses extra oily skin.

Supplements of evening primrose oil and zinc may be helpful.

Stress will also make the skin break out.

NORMAL SKIN CARE

You are very fortunate if you have evenly balanced skin which is smooth, fine-pored, soft and supple, with no spots or blemishes. Children usually have this type of skin, whereas the rest of us have to work hard to achieve it.

There will always be times when this fine balance is disrupted – hormonal problems, illness and erratic diet can disturb the equilibrium.

Although normal skin needs no special extensive care it needs to be well looked after. Wash normal skin with a mild acid or pH-balanced soap daily in warm water. Apply a face mask once a week to ensure that the skin remains evenly balanced.

Face mask for normal skin
2 tablespoons of clay/fuller's earth
1 teaspoon honey
1 teaspoon jojoba or avocado oil
1 drop rose
1 drop geranium or palmarosa

Mix the above ingredients to a thick paste. Apply to the face, avoiding the eye area. Relax ... Leave this mask on until it has dried. Then, gently wash it off with warm water. Use once weekly.

Normal skin should be treated with a facial oil at least once daily to stimulate and nourish the skin.

Normal skin base oils: **sweet almond, apricot kernel, jojoba, peach kernel, evening primrose** and **carrot oil** are all suitable.

Essential oils for normal skin: **German/Roman chamomile, frankincense, geranium, lavender, neroli, palmarosa, rose, rosewood.**

Suggested recipes for normal skin facial oils
Select any of the essential oils from the list above and add them to
your chosen carrier oil(s). The following recipes are useful:

4 drops geranium ⎫
3 drops rose ⎬ or
2 drops rosewood ⎭

3 drops frankincense ⎫ diluted in 30 ml
3 drops lavender ⎬ of carrier oil
3 drops palmarosa ⎭

A facial steambath is also beneficial occasionally. Follow the advice
for oily skin but choose from the essential oils above.

MATURE/AGEING SKIN CARE

As we age, the skin deteriorates and wrinkles appear as the
skin loses its elasticity. Mature skin needs moisture and
oxygen.

....
Insight
The good news is that regular facial aromamassage can do a
great deal to prevent ageing and reduce wrinkling. After just
a few treatments an improvement may be seen. I particularly
recommend carrot seed, frankincense and neroli.
....

Massage stimulates the local circulation and, therefore, brings
good supplies of oxygen to the inner living layers of the skin.
Cell division slows down as we grow older and essential oils
which stimulate cell growth (cytophylactic oils) are indicated.
You can use aromatherapy oils to replace the moisture and treat
dryness.

Anti-ageing base oils: nourishing carrier oils such as **avocado,
jojoba, wheatgerm** and **peach** and **apricot kernel** are excellent for
mature skins.

Essential oils for anti-ageing: **German/Roman chamomile, carrot
seed, clary sage, frankincense, geranium, jasmine, lavender, myrtle,
neroli, palmarosa, rose, yarrow.**

Suggested recipes for ageing skin facial oils
You may select any of the essential oils from the list above and add them to your chosen carrier oil(s). However, you may find the following recipes useful:

3 drops carrot seed			

3 drops carrot seed ⎫
3 drops frankincense ⎬ or
3 drops neroli ⎭

3 drops geranium ⎫
3 drops palmarosa ⎬
3 drops rose ⎭

diluted in
30 ml of
carrier oil

If these oils are to be effective you must apply them to the face daily. Face packs are also worthwhile for mature skins, removing waste products so that cells can be renewed more rapidly.

Face pack for ageing skin
The following recipe is recommended:

2 teaspoons ground almonds
1 teaspoon honey
2 teaspoons water (or rosewater/lavender water)

Mix the ingredients together and add one drop of essential oil of **rose** and one drop of **frankincense**. Apply to the face for 10–15 minutes. Rinse off gently.

Facial steambaths are also useful for mature skin to deep cleanse the pores and stimulate the circulation. Follow the instructions as for oily skin, using two drops of **carrot seed**, two drops of **frankincense** and two drops of **neroli**.

Diet
Adequate nutrition is essential for the skin. Try to consume only small amounts of tea and coffee which help to create the wrinkles and drink two litres of water daily, stop excess consumption of simple sugars, and also eat plenty of fruit and vegetables.

Bee pollen, marine fish extracts, krill oil, Royal Jelly and grapeseed extract all enhance the body's removal of collagen.

Make a smoothie of bio yoghurt, soya or oat milk, berries of choice and capsules of Royal Jelly and krill oil.

Exercise will help to increase the circulation and improve muscle tone. You should avoid extremes of temperature.

ESSENTIAL OILS FOR SKIN PROBLEMS

Acne
Acne occurs primarily during puberty but it can affect people well into their adult years. It is due to overactivity of the sebaceous (oil secreting) glands of the skin. Excessive sebum causes proliferation of bacteria, and the pores become blocked leading to blackheads and spots. It can lead to scarring.

- *Essential oils to clear the body toxins:* **geranium, juniper, lemon, rosemary.**
- *Essential oils to reduce and heal scarring:* **carrot seed, frankincense, lavender, mandarin, neroli.**
- *Essential oils to promote the growth of new cells:* **carrot seed, frankincense, lavender, neroli, palmarosa, patchouli, rosewood.**
- *Essential oils to balance and reduce sebum:* **clary sage, cypress, frankincense, geranium, lavender, lemongrass, yarrow, ylang ylang.**
- *Essential oils as antiseptic and astringent:* **bergamot, cedarwood, myrtle, niaouli, yarrow.**
- *Essential oils to soothe inflammation:* **German/Roman chamomile, yarrow.**

Apply one drop of neat lavender or tea tree undiluted to individual spots. Wash the face with an unscented pH-balanced or acid soap. A facial steambath should be carried out twice a week. Facial oils should be applied daily.

Avoid refined, sweet and fatty foods, smoking, alcohol, tea, coffee and sugary drinks. Plenty of fruit and vegetables are essential as well as lots of water. Vitamin C, zinc and evening primrose oil will help. Exercise is also recommended.

Allergies (e.g. eczema)
Diet, pollutants and stress are all major causes of allergy rashes. It is important to try to identify the allergen – e.g. food, detergents, cosmetics or coarse clothing.

Useful essential oils: **German/Roman chamomile, melissa** and **yarrow** are three of my favourite oils which I use in the treatment of eczema. They certainly seem to reduce itching. Other oils include: **angelica seed, benzoin, geranium, lavender, frankincense, myrrh** and **patchouli** (weeping eczema), **rose otto** and **sandalwood** (dry eczema).

Sometimes carrier oils can make eczema worse, so it is best to blend the essential oils with a non-perfumed organic base cream. The oils can also be applied in cold compresses. Baths are also highly effective.

Athlete's foot
This extremely itchy, infectious fungal condition thrives around and in between the toes. It loves warm and moist conditions.

Useful essential oils: **lavender, myrrh, lemongrass, patchouli** and **tea tree**. Daily footbath using six drops of any of the above oils is recommended. Also dab neat lavender or tea tree on to the affected areas.

Broken capillaries
Weakness in the fine blood vessels can result in the appearance of fine, red veins usually on the cheeks. The capillaries are not really broken but are just weak and stretched. The capillary walls are supposed to be elastic, enlarging when the skin is hot and then shrinking back to their original size. If they lose their elasticity, they are prematurely dilated (enlarged) leading to a ruddy complexion.

Gentle facial massage can help to promote contraction of the blood vessels. Try the following formula over a period of months:

3 drops German/Roman chamomile ⎤
3 drops geranium ⎬ diluted in 30 ml of carrier oil
3 drops rose ⎦

Cypress, frankincense, neroli and patchouli are also useful.

To enhance the treatment, avoid spicy foods, alcohol, smoking, caffeine and stress. Vitamin C is also beneficial.

Cellulite

Cellulite, sometimes referred to as 'orange peel skin', affects women almost exclusively, forming on the thighs, hips and buttocks, and therefore it seems to be hormone related. It is characterized by lymphatic congestion, water retention, an increase in fatty tissue and often poor circulation.

Aromatherapy together with nutritional advice and exercise is quite a successful treatment for cellulite, if you persevere. The aim of the treatment is to stimulate the lymphatic system, balance the hormones and reduce the water retention.

▶ *Essential oils to reduce fluid:* **angelica seed, cypress, fennel, grapefruit, juniper, lemon, lemongrass, lime, pine, rosemary** *and* **sandalwood.**
▶ *Essential oils to stimulate the circulatory and detoxify the lymphatic systems:* **angelica seed, benzoin, black pepper, cardamom, carrot seed, cedarwood, coriander, cypress, fennel, ginger, patchouli, pine, rosemary, sage.**
▶ *Essential oils to balance the hormones:* **German/Roman chamomile, clary sage, geranium, lavender** *and* **rose.**

ACTION PLAN FOR CELLULITE

1 *Dry skin brushing daily. Brush in upward movements all over the body with a natural hair bristle brush, paying particular*

attention to the affected areas. This will detoxify and improve the circulation.

2 *Bathe at least once a day, choosing from the oils above or using one of the following formulae:*

3 drops cypress 3 drops fennel 3 drops juniper berry	or	3 drops black pepper 3 drops lemon 3 drops grapefruit	or	3 drops geranium 3 drops fennel 3 drops rose	diluted in 30 ml of carrier oil

Follow the bath with a cold shower.

3 *Massage the affected area twice daily – morning and evening – using the following formulae:*

3 drops fennel 3 drops grapefruit 3 drops lemon	or	3 drops cypress 3 drops geranium 3 drops juniper berry	diluted in 30 ml of carrier oil

4 *Pay attention to your diet. Eliminate tea, coffee and alcohol. Drink only spring water and herb teas – fennel tea is excellent. Hot water and lemon first thing in the morning and before bed is very cleansing. Eat plenty of fresh fruit and vegetables (raw if possible). Avoid sugar and refined carbohydrates as well as salty food. Avoid dairy foods from cows. Increase your vitamin C intake to at least 1 g daily. Guto Kola extract applied topically alleviates cellulitis.*

5 *Exercise daily for about 20 minutes – swimming and cycling are perfect.*

6 *Relaxation is vital as stress can affect the hormonal balance and elimination is less efficient.*

Cold sores (herpes)
Cold sores are the result of lowered immunity, stress, extremes of temperature and excessively strong sunlight. They are caused

by the herpes simplex virus. It is important to apply the essential oils at the first sign of an eruption. Dip a cotton bud into either of the following solutions and dab several times a day:

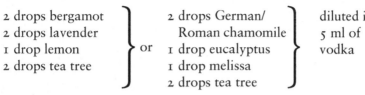

2 drops bergamot		2 drops German/		diluted in
2 drops lavender		Roman chamomile		5 ml of
1 drop lemon	or	1 drop eucalyptus		vodka
2 drops tea tree		1 drop melissa		
		2 drops tea tree		

Neat lavender or tea tree oil can also be used on the blisters. Take at least 1g of vitamin C daily and 1000 mg of lysine and B complex. Eat plenty of fruit and vegetables and wholegrains.

Infectious skin conditions
Conditions such as chickenpox, scabies and measles should never be massaged when presented by a client. Use six drops of any of the following oils in the bath: **bergamot, lavender, lemon, ravensara, rosemary, tea tree.**

Psoriasis
This condition is characterized by the formulation of red patches which are covered by scaly skin, occurring mostly on the elbows, knees, palms of the hands, soles of the feet and on the head. Psoriasis is often inherited but may not appear until adulthood. The cause is unknown, although stress appears to be a major factor.

Psoriasis is a difficult condition to treat but it usually responds to aromatherapy.

Essential oils for psoriasis: **benzoin, bergamot, cajeput, German/Roman chamomile, lavender, niaouli and yarrow.** Any of the above oils may be blended with a carrier oil or mixed into a pure organic skin cream (see page 32 for details of creams).

SUGGESTED RECIPES FOR PSORIASIS
Select any of the essential oils from the list above and add them to
your chosen carrier oil(s). The following recipes are useful:

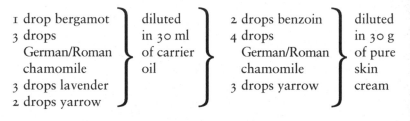

1 drop bergamot
3 drops
   German/Roman
   chamomile
3 drops lavender
2 drops yarrow
} diluted
in 30 ml
of carrier
oil

2 drops benzoin
4 drops
   German/Roman
   chamomile
3 drops yarrow
} diluted
in 30 g
of pure
skin
cream

DIET
Avoid smoking and drinking alcohol and coffee. Drinking fruit juices
and two litres of water daily is beneficial. Fruit and vegetables (raw
if possible) and simple wholefoods are recommended. Carrot, garlic,
onion, rhubarb and tomatoes are particularly beneficial. Eat oily fish
such as mackerel, sardines and tuna. Vitamins A, B complex, B_{12}, C,
E, zinc, selenium, curcumin, coenzyme (improved immune function
of skin) and evening primrose oil may also be helpful. Juicing and
sprouting are beneficial.

Moderate sun can also help psoriasis. Never wear unnatural fibres
such as polyester or nylon next to the skin.

Hair

Just as our skin is a reflection of our inner health, so is our hair.
The condition of our hair is, to a large extent, dependent on
optimum health and nutrition. Hormonal changes, hereditary
factors, stress, overexposure to ultraviolet rays, chemicals such as
perms, dyes and hairsprays, pollutants and drugs will all affect the
health of our hair. The health of our hair also depends upon the
way that we treat it. It is vital that the hair is brushed thoroughly,
preferably not with a nylon brush, to remove the old dead hair
and stimulate natural growth. We have approximately 100,000
hairs on the scalp. Blondes have the most hair and the finest hair

in comparison to redheads who have the least hair and the coarsest hair. Every day approximately 80 hairs are lost!

Insight

My grandmother used to tell me to brush my hair 100 times a day and she was right; brushing massages the scalp, stimulates the circulation and removes old hair.

Essential oils are valuable in hair care because they can influence and balance the sebaceous glands. The sebum which is secreted by these glands lubricates and protects the hair. If these glands are sluggish and underactive the hair will become dry and dehydrated. Conversely, if the sebaceous glands are overactive, the hair will become oily. Essential oils are beneficial to all types of hair for regulating the production of sebum.

WASHING THE HAIR

Many commercial shampoos contain chemical and synthetic substances which damage the scalp and the hair follicles. They attack the acid mantle of the scalp and wash away the hair's natural protective oils. Therefore, after each washing the hair should be rinsed with an acidic substance such as lemon juice or organic apple cider vinegar. This will wash out any residues of soap and will help to restore the acid equilibrium of the scalp.

You should avoid using the harsh detergent-based shampoos. Choose a mild natural shampoo which will be less likely to disturb the acid mantle of the scalp.

Insight

Make your own shampoo using the following recipe:

100 g soap flakes (available from some health shops and pharmacies)

1 litre spring water

(Contd)

1 Simmer the spring water and add soap flakes, stirring until the flakes dissolve. Allow the mixture to cool and pour into a bottle or jar.
2 Add essential oils to this shampoo base, depending on your hair type.

NORMAL HAIR (HEALTHY HAIR)

Normal hair is neither too dry nor too greasy, easy to comb, strong, self-renewing and shining. The following essential oils are useful to keep the hair healthy.

Essential oils for normal hair: **German/Roman chamomile, carrot seed, geranium, lavender, lemon, rosemary, rosewood.**

Insight
The chamomiles and lemon are particularly effective for light hair. Carrot seed is good for ginger hair and rosemary and rosewood will enhance dark hair.

Suggested recipes for normal hair shampoo
Select any of the essential oils from the list above and add them to your shampoo base. You will find the following recipes useful:

Blonde hair	Dark hair	
8 drops German/ Roman chamomile	8 drops lemon	Mix together with 100 ml shampoo base, and bottle
8 drops carrot seed	8 drops carrot seed	
8 drops geranium	or 8 drops rosemary	
8 drops lemon	8 drops rosewood	

Rinse for normal hair
1 cup of water
1 teaspoon of cider vinegar
3 drops lemon (blonde hair) or
3 drops rosemary (dark hair)

Deep, normal hair conditioning treatment and recipes
Once a week normal hair should be nourished with a deep
conditioning hair treatment, particularly if it is washed
frequently or has been exposed to the sun, wind or chlorine
in the swimming pool.

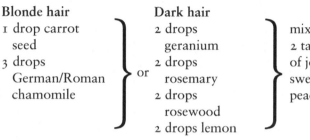

Blonde hair
1 drop carrot
   seed
3 drops
   German/Roman
   chamomile

or

Dark hair
2 drops
   geranium
2 drops
   rosemary
2 drops
   rosewood
2 drops lemon

mixed with
2 tablespoons
of jojoba oil/
sweet almond oil/
peach kernel

Massage the oil thoroughly into the hair and then cover the head
with a plastic shower cap. Leave the oil on the head for two hours
or even overnight. Shampoo the hair as usual.

DRY HAIR

Dry hair is caused by the inactivity of the sebaceous glands.
Aromatherapy treatment is directed towards stimulating the
glands to restore the hair to its natural condition. Essential
oils for dry hair: **carrot seed, German/Roman chamomile,
geranium, lavender, palmarosa, rosewood, sandalwood,
ylang ylang.**

Insight
Dry hair should always be protected from the sun,
sea and swimming pools which can only aggravate
the condition.

Suggested recipes for dry hair shampoo
Select any of the essential oils from the list above and add them to
the shampoo base.

You will find the following recipes useful:

8 drops carrot seed 8 drops lavender 8 drops palmarosa 8 drops ylang ylang	or	8 drops geranium 8 drops parsley 8 drops sandalwood 8 drops ylang ylang	Blend well with 100 ml shampoo base and 1 teaspoon of jojoba/avocado/peach kernel carrier oil, and bottle

Rinse for dry hair
1 cup of water
1 teaspoon of cider vinegar
3 drops sandalwood *or*
3 drops ylang ylang

Blend the above ingredients well and add to the bowl of water you are using as your final rinse. Immerse your hair thoroughly.

Deep dry hair conditioning treatment and recipe
It is essential to nourish dry hair, which has often been damaged by bleach and other chemicals as well as by the elements. Jojoba oil is particularly effective against dry, brittle hair and split ends. The following recipe is recommended and should be used at least once a week:

2 tablespoons jojoba oil
1 drop carrot seed
2 drops geranium
2 drops ylang ylang

Apply the above oil all over the scalp. Massage thoroughly and cover the hair with a plastic shower cap or polythene bag. Leave on for at least two hours or even overnight, then shampoo and rinse as usual.

OILY HAIR

Oily hair is caused by an overactivity of the sebaceous glands.

> **Insight**
>
> Oily hair is exacerbated by shampooing too often with commercial shampoo, and the more you wash with these products the worse the condition becomes. If you use a mild shampoo then it is perfectly acceptable to wash it every day.

Essential oils for oily hair: **bergamot, cedarwood, clary sage, cypress, frankincense, juniper, lavender, lemon, niaouli, rosemary, sage, thyme, yarrow.**

Suggested recipe for oily hair shampoo
Select any of the essential oils from the list above and add them to the shampoo base. You will find the following recipe useful:

8 drops cedarwood	Blend well with 100 ml of
8 drops clary sage	shampoo base, and bottle
8 drops cypress	
8 drops lemon	

Rinse for oily hair
1 cup of water
2 teaspoon of cider vinegar (or lemon juice)
2 drops lemon
1 drop thyme

Blend the above ingredients well and add to your final rinse, ensuring that the whole scalp is effectively treated.

Hair tonic for oily hair
A hair tonic is particularly effective for oily hair. It should be massaged into the hair and left on overnight. This treatment should be carried out at least once a week and, if the condition is severe, two or three times.

2 cups of spring water (or boiled water)
2 tablespoons of apple cider vinegar/fresh lemon juice
2 drops bergamot

2 drops clary sage
3 drops cypress
2 drops lavender
1 drop thyme

Blend well and bottle. Rub into the scalp.

Deep oily hair conditioning recipe and treatment
Oily hair needs to be conditioned about once a week.

2 tablespoons sweet almond oil
2 drops bergamot
2 drops cypress
2 drops lemon
2 drops yarrow

Blend the ingredients together and thoroughly massage the conditioner into the scalp. Cover the hair with a plastic shower cap or polythene bag. Leave for 15 minutes. Then shampoo and rinse as usual.

DIET

Your hair reacts to the foods that you eat. Your diet provides you with all the necessary vitamins and minerals for a healthy head of hair, full of lustre. Avoid coffee, tea, alcohol, smoking, saturated fats and sugar. Eat plenty of fresh fruit and vegetables and unsaturated fatty acids. Eggs and kelp improve the condition of hair as do nettle and parsley juice. Chestnuts and flax seed oil are also beneficial.

Protect your hair as much as possible from strong sunlight, sea and chlorinated swimming pools. If you are going down to the beach for the day, why not apply a deep conditioning treatment? The warmth from the sun will enhance the effects of the treatment.

Try to relax as much as possible as stress and tension can actually make you lose your hair.

ESSENTIAL OILS FOR OTHER HAIR PROBLEMS

Dandruff
Basil, carrot seed, German/Roman chamomile, cypress, eucalyptus, patchouli, peppermint, rosemary and thyme are all beneficial for dandruff. Use them in your shampoo, rinses and hair oils. Always ensure that you rinse your hair thoroughly.

Hair loss
The following essential oils should be mixed into your hair products to stimulate hair growth: basil, German/Roman chamomile, cedarwood, clary sage, cypress, frankincense, geranium, ginger, lavender, peppermint, rosemary, thyme and yarrow.

Head lice
As a mother of two children I have lots of experience in dealing with these. I have found the following essential oils to be effective: bergamot, eucalyptus, geranium, lavender, lemon, niaouli, rosemary and tea tree.

Most children are unfortunately likely to pick up head lice at least once in their schooldays. Essential oils added to shampoos are a good preventive treatment. Also add one drop of rosemary and one drop of tea tree to the final rinse.

LICE TREATMENT FOR CHILDREN

2 tablespoons of carrier oil
1 drop lavender
1 drop lemon
1 drop rosemary
1 drop tea tree

Blend the ingredients together well, apply to the hair, cover with a polythene shower cap and leave overnight for maximum benefit. Comb through the hair thoroughly with a fine-toothed 'nit comb', available from chemists, to remove lice and eggs. Shampoo and rinse as usual.

Never be embarrassed if your child has head lice. All children are vulnerable.

TEST YOUR KNOWLEDGE

1 *In cases of dry skin are the sebaceous glands underactive or overactive?*

2 *You are making up a 30 ml facial blend – how many drops of essential oil are required?*

3 *Which three essential oils in the following list are suitable for dry skin? Carrot seed, cypress, lemon, rose, rosemary, sandalwood*

4 *Why should cosmetics containing alcohol be avoided if you have dry skin?*

5 *In cases of oily skin are the sebaceous glands producing too much or too little sebum?*

6 *At what stage of life is oily skin most common?*

7 *Chose two essential oils beneficial for oily skin. Bergamot, chamomile, lemon, sandalwood*

8 *Choose two essential oils useful for rejuvenation and ageing skin. Peppermint, rose, frankincense, lemon*

9 *Which two essential oils may be applied undiluted to individual spots?*

10 *Name one essential oil particularly suitable for:*
   a *blonde hair*
   b *ginger hair*
   c *dark hair*

13

Women's problems

In this chapter you will learn:
- *the causes and effects of the most common female problems*
- *the orthodox treatment that is prescribed*
- *which essential oils to use for 'women's problems'*
- *which Bach Flower Remedies to take*
- *simple dietary and lifestyle changes to use alongside your aromatherapy treatment.*

Women can be unfortunate enough to suffer from a host of problems. In this chapter I have covered premenstrual syndrome (PMS) and menopausal problems in detail as these are the two most common disorders that seem to present themselves at my clinic. I have covered the other 'women's problems' more briefly.

If your problem is severe or prolonged, please go to a gynaecologist to ensure that you do not have a serious medical condition.

Amenorrhoea (absence of periods)

Amenorrhoea is the absence or loss of periods and it can be brought on by a number of factors, such as anorexia, slimming diets, strenuous physical training (e.g. athletics, gymnastics), disease of the ovaries or even coming off the contraceptive pill.

Emotional upsets such as stress, shock and rapid changes can also result in amenorrhoea.

ORTHODOX TREATMENT

The cause of the amenorrhoea should always be identified. If the cause is an ovarian cyst this will be surgically removed and anorexia will require specialist treatment too. Hormone treatment may be given to induce ovulation.

AROMATHERAPY TREATMENT

If the problems are due to an emotional source, it should resolve itself in time. However, there are essential oils which encourage the menstrual cycle to re-establish itself again.

Useful oils include: **basil, carrot seed, German/Roman chamomile, clary sage, cypress, geranium, fennel, hyssop, juniper, marjoram, myrrh, niaouli, peppermint, rose, rosemary** and **thyme.**

Baths
Choose any combination of the above oils and put six drops into your daily bath.

Insight
Why not try a sitz bath? I recommend adding two drops clary sage, two drops cypress and two drops rose to a bowl of hand-hot water or bidet and sitting in it for approximately 10 minutes.

Aromamassage
The following combination(s) of essential oils should be massaged into your abdomen and your low back daily for about a month:

2 drops cypress
2 drops fennel
1 drop juniper berry
1 drop marjoram

or

1 drop carrot seed
3 drops geranium
2 drops rose

diluted in
20 ml of
carrier oil

It is beneficial to have a full body aromatherapy massage with either of the suggested blends on a weekly basis if stress has induced the amenorrhoea.

Contraindications
Do not use **fennel** excessively in case of epilepsy. **Thyme** may increase the blood pressure.

BACH FLOWER REMEDIES

The Remedy **Star of Bethlehem** is excellent for shock. Stressful situations also call for **Rescue Remedy**. Amenorrhoea caused by anorexia will require several remedies depending upon the individual – **Mimulus** is needed where there is a great fear (e.g. fear of getting fat), **Crab Apple** will help to cleanse away feelings of self-disgust and is for those who find food abhorrent, **Beech** is excellent for those who are self-critical, **Pine** is indicated for guilt and **Agrimony** for inner torture.

DIET

A healthy diet is essential to resolve problems of amenorrhoea. A gentle cleansing diet with broths and soups will help initially. Avoid all processed foods and junk foods. Oily fish or essential fatty acid supplements are beneficial and chasteberry alleviates two-thirds of cases. Black cohosh and liquorice root may be useful. Drink chamomile tea and beetroot juice.

Try steeping tea of chamomile, liquorice root with chasteberry (loose herbs or tincture).

Dysmenorrhoea (painful periods)

Dysmenorrhoea, or painful periods, is a relatively common problem and the symptoms can vary from a slight ache to a violent cramping sensation that causes you to keel over and take to your bed. It is caused by cramp of the uterine muscles. There are two types of dysmenorrhoea – spasmodic cramping, a sharp pain often appearing on the first day of menstruation, and congestive cramping, a dull aching pain which usually starts prior to menstruation.

ORTHODOX TREATMENT

Dysmenorrhoea can usually be relieved by taking analgesic drugs (painkillers) such as aspirin. If pain is severe, oral contraceptives may be prescribed to suppress ovulation.

AROMATHERAPY TREATMENT

Useful oils include: **angelica seed, German/Roman chamomile, cajeput, clary sage, cypress, fennel, ginger, jasmine, juniper, lavender, marjoram, melissa, niaouli, peppermint, rose** and **rosemary.**

Baths
You may experiment with different formulae to find the right combination for you.

Insight
One of my favourite recipes for the bath for painful menstruation is two drops German/Roman chamomile, two drops clary sage and two drops marjoram. This formula is excellent for relieving cramping.

Compresses
Aromatherapy compresses are one of the most effective ways of affording relief from menstrual pain. You may try any one of the oils from the list since they are all antispasmodic. **Lavender** and **peppermint** are an excellent combination (three drops each) as are **German/Roman chamomile** and **marjoram. Clary sage** and **rose** can also be used.

Aromamassage
This is particularly effective when performed on the abdomen or the low back area. Sometimes osteopathic treatment can bring

relief from dysmenorrhoea. Massage the abdomen daily with one of the following blends:

2 drops clary sage			2 drops fennel		diluted in
1 drop cypress	}	or	1 drop juniper berry	}	20 ml of
2 drops marjoram			2 drops peppermint		carrier oil
1 drop rose			1 drop sage		

Contraindications
Avoid excessive use of **fennel** in cases of epilepsy.

BACH FLOWER REMEDIES

Rescue Remedy may be useful for pain relief. **Crab Apple** is recommended where there is congestion.

DIET

A healthy diet is essential with plenty of fruit and vegetables, cutting out sugar and refined foods. Useful supplements include evening primrose oil, calcium, magnesium, vitamin B complex and vitamin E.

Blackberry juice, ginger, raspberry leaf and passion flower and angelica (regulates muscular activity in uterus) are all beneficial.

Increase your oily fish intake or take a supplement.

Endometriosis

This is a condition whereby clumps of endometrial cells which normally line the uterus (the endometrium) appear and grow outside the uterus such as in the ovaries, Fallopian tubes, the bladder, intestines, lungs and elsewhere. It is still not clear how this problem develops.

SYMPTOMS

Endometriosis affects at least 1 million women in this
country – I say 'at least' as many cases of endometriosis remain
undiagnosed for years. It is surprising that so little is written
about it! Although the symptoms are variable they include painful
periods, pain on ovulation and intercourse, heavy bleeding,
erratic bleeding, pain when emptying the bowels or passing
water, infertility, nausea, anxiety and depression. The pain can be
absolutely excruciating with the sufferer rolling around the floor
in agony.

TREATMENT

Orthodox treatment
Drugs such as danazol, a testosterone drug which has many
unpleasant side-effects, are prescribed. A laparoscopy may be
performed in order to examine the abdomen. Sometimes surgery
is necessary.

Aromatherapy treatment
Aromatherapy is helpful in some cases for relieving the pain
and to relax the sufferer. Stress undoubtedly makes the pain
much worse.

Useful oils include: **bergamot, German/Roman chamomile, cypress,
geranium, lavender, peppermint, rose** and **yarrow**.

Sitz baths
Although aromatherapy baths are relaxing, hot and cold sitz baths
are particularly recommended for endometriosis. The aim of this
treatment is to encourage the blood vessels to contract and to
dilate. You will need two washing-up bowls for this method
(baby baths are ideal, too). Fill up one bowl with hot water and
one with cold water. Sit in the hot sitz bath for ten minutes and
then in the cold sitz bath for five minutes. Repeat this procedure
two or three times (you may need to add some more hot water
to the hot bath).

The following blend should be added to the hot bath only:

1 drop German/Roman chamomile
1 drop clary sage
2 drops cypress
1 drop geranium
1 drop rose

The hot and cold sitz baths should be carried out daily. If you find this method impossible then add the blend to your bath instead.

Aromamassage

Massage the abdomen and the low back area every day using one of the following formulae:

2 drops German/Roman chamomile 2 drops cypress 2 drops yarrow	or 2 drops clary sage 3 drops geranium 1 drop rose	diluted in 20 ml of carrier oil

In order to get results the aromatherapy baths and daily massages should be carried out for several months. Do persevere!

Compresses

Alternate hot or cold compresses may be used to provide pain relief. **Peppermint, clary sage** and **lavender** are probably the most effective essential oils. Into a small bowl of water put two drops of clary sage, two drops of lavender and two drops of peppermint. Soak up the solution on to your flannel, squeeze it out and place it on to the abdomen or lower back area – wherever the pain is most severe.

A peppermint compress will also be useful in cases of nausea.

Contraindications

Do not use **fennel** excessively in cases of epilepsy. Avoid **peppermint** if taking homoeopathic medication.

BACH FLOWER REMEDIES

To ease the physical and emotional tension it is well worth trying some **Rescue Remedy**.

DIET

A healthy diet, exercise and relaxation should also be followed by those with endometriosis. Avoid stress as much as possible. Evening primrose oil can help to relieve the pain and cramping. Natural progesterone is proven to be helpful. Black cohosh, chasteberry and grapeseed extract are beneficial.

Gentle cleansing broths and soups are easily digested and comforting. Increase fish oils and EPA (eicosapentaenoic acid) as these reportedly reduce the area of the endometrium affected by the endometriosis.

Menopause

The menopause usually occurs somewhere between the ages of 45 and 55 and means the end of the monthly menstruation cycle. Although some women stop menstruating abruptly, most women experience an erratic cycle for several years prior to the cessation of menstruating. It is a gradual process. Nowadays many people regard the menopause as an illness when in fact it is a normal state of a woman's development.

SYMPTOMS

The most commonly experienced symptoms include hot flushes, heavy night sweating, irregular periods with scanty or heavy bleeding (flooding), dizziness and fainting, irritability, insomnia, depression, memory loss, headaches, constipation and weight gain, cold hands and feet, and increased or reduced libido. Blood pressure also rises after the menopause, vaginal dryness can occur and some women experience hair loss.

It is interesting that women who are stressed or who lead a physically and sexually inactive life have far more problems in the menopause.

TREATMENT

Orthodox treatment
Consists of hormone replacement therapy (HRT). Although this treatment increases bone density – but only when you are taking it – it does have side-effects. It can lead to hypertension, weight gain and has been linked with an increased risk of cancer of the breast and uterus. More research is needed to investigate possible side-effects.

Aromatherapy treatment
Although all women will have a different experience of the menopause I have found the following essential oils to be helpful with my clients: **bergamot, German/Roman chamomile, clary sage, cypress, fennel, frankincense, geranium, jasmine, juniper, lavender, lemon, melissa, neroli, peppermint, rose, rosemary, sandalwood, yarrow** and **ylang ylang**.

Insight
My advice is to try essential oils, which can have a remarkable effect on the regulation of hormones. Aromatherapy coupled with the right diet and an exercise programme can offer an alternative to HRT. The menopause should be approached in a positive way instead of with feelings of dread.

On an emotional level there are many essential oils which can help to alleviate the depression and irritability of the menopause. Bergamot is a wonderfully uplifting oil as is clary sage which can induce a sense of well-being. Chamomile is important for relieving the nervous tension associated with the menopause. Cypress not only relieves irritability and stress but is also highly effective for times of change, easing the transition.

The menopause, of course, is often referred to as 'the change'. Frankincense will enable a woman to move on and enjoy the freedom and exhilaration that the menopause can offer. Geranium is sedative yet uplifting and is also a balancer of the hormones and the skin. The exquisite aromas of jasmine, neroli and rose cannot fail to lift depression and induce optimism, euphoria and confidence.

On a physical level there are essential oils which will deal with the uncomfortable and embarrassing hot flushes caused by the irregular function of the blood vessels as they contract and dilate. Peppermint, cypress, clary sage, geranium and lemon are all useful for these symptoms. To counteract fluid retention, bloating and constipation, cypress, fennel, geranium, juniper, lemon and rosemary may be applied. Insomnia may be relieved by putting a few drops of clary sage, chamomile, lavender or ylang ylang on your pillow. Chamomile, geranium, rose and yarrow are often employed to regulate the menstrual cycle. To help with circulation geranium, peppermint and rosemary are beneficial.

Baths
Daily aromatherapy baths are an enormous help as you go through the menopause. Try some of the following blends or choose from my list.

Nerve balancing formulae
2 drops German/Roman chamomile
2 drops cypress
2 drops rose

or

2 drops clary sage
2 drops frankincense
2 drops lavender

Hot flushes formula
3 drops cypress
3 drops peppermint

Bloated/constipation formula
2 drops fennel
2 drops rosemary
2 drops cardamom

Aromamassage

Aromamassage is an excellent way of pampering and nurturing a woman as she goes through 'the change'. It increases self-esteem and can make her feel positive, confident and feminine. It is excellent for minimizing the physical problems, too. Try the following formulae:

Uplifting formulae

2 drops bergamot
1 drop German/
   Roman chamomile
1 drop cypress
2 drops rose
} or

2 drops frankincense
2 drops geranium
1 drop jasmine
1 drop melissa
} diluted in 20 ml of carrier oil

Hot flushes/sweating formula

2 drops cypress
2 drops lemon
2 drops peppermint
} diluted in 20 ml of carrier oil

....

Insight

For emergencies you may like to keep a bottle of essential oil of geranium or peppermint in your handbag and inhale to help with hot flushes.

....

Cold hands and feet formula

1 drop black pepper
1 drop mandarin
2 drops geranium
2 drops rosemary
} diluted in 20 ml of carrier oil

Fluid retention/bloatedness formula

2 drops cypress
1 drop mandarin
2 drops juniper berry
1 drop rosemary
} diluted in 20 ml of carrier oil

For formulae for vaginal dryness, and loss of libido please refer to Chapter 15. For hair loss and skin problems refer to Chapter 12. For poor circulation and high blood pressure refer to Chapter 9.

Insight

If you find that you are suffering from confusion and a poor memory, try inhaling a few drops of rosemary from a tissue several times a day.

Contraindications

Avoid excessive use of **fennel** if you are epileptic. Do not apply **bergamot** and **lemon** before sunbathing. Avoid **peppermint** when taking homoeopathic medications.

BACH FLOWER REMEDIES

Walnut is the most important Remedy during the menopause as it assists 'change'. **Larch** is excellent for restoring confidence. For feelings of hopelessness and despair try **Gorse**. For mood swings and indecision **Scleranthus** can be very helpful. Use **Impatiens** for irritability and **Willow** for resentment. **Olive** is essential for fatigue and tiredness.

DIET

Diet is important during the menopause if osteoporosis is to be prevented. Calcium-rich foods should be increased to maintain strong and healthy bones. These include fish such as sardines, where the bones are eaten, sunflower, pumpkin and sesame seeds, nuts and dairy foods if they can be tolerated. Since calcium requires vitamin D in order to be absorbed it is vital to go out into the sunshine. Exercise – especially skipping or jumping on the spot – can increase your bone density.

As calorie needs decline with the onset of the menopause you must eat less. Avoid salt and refined sugar. Reduce tea, coffee and alcohol intake. Increase your intake of fruit, vegetables and fibre. Try vitamin C

(1 g daily) and evening primrose oil for the hot flushes. Take an iron supplement to counteract blood loss if there is 'flooding' and vitamin B complex, zinc, vitamin C, calcium and magnesium for stress. Calcium and magnesium are also vital for preventing the loss of bone.

Aniseed tea, black cohosh, chasteberry and wild yam are also beneficial in reducing symptoms.

Relaxation is important – aromatherapy baths and massage are ideal. Remember also to think positively.

Menorrhagia (heavy bleeding)

Menorrhagia is profuse bleeding often with clotting. Abnormally heavy bleeding can occur at any time during a woman's life, but it is particularly common around the time of the menopause.

Insight
Profuse bleeding or bleeding between periods should always be diagnosed by a medically qualified doctor to ensure that there is no serious medical condition.

ORTHODOX TREATMENT

If the woman is young, hormones may be prescribed to reduce the amount of bleeding. Otherwise a D and C (dilation and curettage) may be carried out or if the condition is severe a hysterectomy (removal of the uterus) may be performed.

AROMATHERAPY TREATMENT

Once the menorrhagia has been checked out, aromatherapy treatment can begin with the aim of regulating the periods.

Useful oils include: **German/Roman chamomile, cypress, frankincense, geranium, juniper, lemon, rose** and **yarrow**.

Baths/sitz baths
Any of the essential oils above may be added to your bath or in a sitz bath.

3 drops geranium 3 drops lemon	2 drops cypress 2 drops frankincense 2 drops yarrow	or	3 drops juniper berry 3 drops lemon

Use this formula when the womb needs cleansing.

Aromamassage
The abdomen and lower back can be massaged gently every day with one of the following blends:

2 drops German/Roman chamomile 1 drop frankincense 2 drops geranium 1 drop yarrow	or	2 drops cypress 2 drops lemon 2 drops rose	diluted in 20 ml of carrier oil

Contraindications
Avoid **lemon** prior to sunbathing.

BACH FLOWER REMEDIES

Crab Apple is indicated if cleansing is required. Use **Rescue Remedy** to provide pain relief.

DIET

A healthy diet is essential. It should be remembered that heavy periods can result in iron deficiency (anaemia). Please refer to pages 196–99 for details on this condition. Menorrhagia can also be caused by chronic iron deficiency. Kelp can correct profuse bleeding caused by a thyroid deficiency and increase folic acid, vitamin A, vitamin B_{12} and vitamin C. Ground chestnuts alleviate abnormally heavy bleeding associated with menorrhagia.

Premenstrual syndrome (PMS)

The above term is used to describe the wide range of symptoms which affect women in the second half of the menstrual cycle. Women can be affected anything from three days to two weeks prior to menstruation.

SYMPTOMS

Over 150 symptoms have been attributed to PMS, although most women thankfully will suffer from just a few of them. The most common physical and psychological symptoms include:

▶ *anxiety, irritability and mood swings*
▶ *bloating of the abdomen*
▶ *breast tenderness*
▶ *fatigue, fainting and dizziness*
▶ *feelings of aggression, violence and suicide*
▶ *fluid retention*
▶ *headaches and migraine*
▶ *increased appetite and cravings for sweet things*
▶ *lack of concentration, confusion, clumsiness and forgetfulness*
▶ *skin problems*
▶ *weight gain.*

In Western societies there has been a vast increase in PMS.

TREATMENT

Orthodox treatment
May involve taking the contraceptive pill and drugs to relieve anxiety. Some doctors now recommend supplements such as evening primrose oil.

Aromatherapy treatment
Aromatherapy is highly effective and it has helped enormous numbers of sufferers to overcome this distressing condition.

When selecting your essential oils, both the physical and emotional problems should be addressed. For maximum benefit, it is vital that the oils are used alongside a nutritional programme.

Every woman has a different experience of PMS and, therefore, it is impossible to provide one solution for this hormonal imbalance. However, the following essential oils have been found to be successful: **benzoin, bergamot, carrot seed, cedarwood, German/Roman chamomile, clary sage, cypress, fennel, frankincense, geranium, grapefruit, jasmine, juniper, lemon, melissa, neroli, rose, rosemary, sandalwood** and **ylang ylang**.

On an emotional level there are many essential oils that can help to reduce anxiety and uplift depression. Benzoin is renowned for its warming effects on the emotions and bergamot is effective for alleviating depression. Cedarwood calms and soothes nervous states and carrot seed relieves tension and exhaustion. The chamomiles ease anger and irritability and balance mood swings. Clary sage is a wonderful euphoric-sedative oil which can calm an overactive mind inducing feelings of optimism. Cypress is a comforting oil ideal for relieving states of anger and irritability. Frankincense instils feelings of calmness and serenity and geranium balances the nervous system. Grapefruit is refreshing and reviving for a listless, apathetic state of mind. Jasmine is a marvellous oil for uplifting depression encouraging positive thoughts and actions. Melissa is soothing and calming, dispelling melancholy, and neroli is advantageous for bringing peace and tranquillity to an agitated mind. Palmarosa helps to raise a low self-esteem and parsley soothes and calms aggression. Rose exerts a profound effect on the emotions and is recommended for particularly difficult cases. Sandalwood and ylang ylang are deeply relaxing, releasing anger and tension.

On a physical level cypress, fennel, geranium, juniper, lemon and rosemary are excellent oils to help to minimize or completely eradicate fluid retention. They are all excellent detoxifiers.

Breast tenderness can be soothed by oils such as German/Roman chamomile, cypress, geranium and rose.

Headaches may be calmed and soothed with compresses of German/Roman chamomile, peppermint and lavender.

Insight

Fennel is one of the most effective oils for helping to balance the appetite and will, therefore, help to reduce the cravings for cakes, chocolate and sweets which is so characteristic of PMS. It will also prevent weight gain.

Baths

Aromatherapy baths should be taken on a daily basis. The following blends may be helpful but, as usual, I urge you to select your oils from the list until you find a combination which absolutely suits you:

Fluid retention formulae

2 drops cypress
2 drops fennel
2 drops juniper berry
} or
2 drops geranium
2 drops lemon
2 drops rosemary
}

Anger/irritability formulae

2 drops German/Roman chamomile
2 drops geranium
2 drops ylang ylang
} or
2 drops bergamot
3 drops palmarosa
1 drop lavender
}

Depression formulae

2 drops bergamot
3 drops clary sage
1 drop rose
} or
2 drops cedarwood
2 drops jasmine
2 drops melissa
}

Fatigue formulae

2 drops carrot seed
2 drops grapefruit
2 drops lemon
} or
3 drops lemon
2 drops rosemary
1 drop lime
}

Aromamassage

Aromamassage, especially lymphatic drainage techniques, can assist enormously with fluid retention. A full body massage should be carried out a day or two prior to the onset of the fluid retention. Self-massage of the affected areas is also highly recommended.

Massage is also the best method of reducing the psychological symptoms. It gives the woman some time to relax and unwind, to get things into proportion once again. The following blends are useful:

Fluid retention formula

2 drops cypress   } diluted in 20 ml of
1 drop geranium   } carrier oil
2 drops juniper berry   }
1 drop rosemary   }

Anxiety/mood swing formulae

3 drops German/		2 drops bergamot		diluted in
Roman chamomile	or	2 drops clary sage		20 ml of
1 drop palmarosa		1 drop geranium		carrier oil
2 drops rose		1 drop rose		

....

Insight

> A combination of massage at least once a month and daily aromatherapy baths is the best way to combat PMS. For a quick fix you can inhale a few drops of essential oil from a handkerchief – this can have a profound effect on the nervous system. Carry a bottle of geranium or the more luxurious rose oil around with you.

....

Contraindications

Avoid **fennel** excessively in epilepsy. **Bergamot, grapefruit** and **lemon** should not be applied prior to sunbathing.

BACH FLOWER REMEDIES

Walnut is an excellent remedy to use throughout the menstrual cycle as it is indicated for adjustments and change and this is what the menstrual cycle is. **Impatiens** should be used for anger, irritability and impatience, which are all major symptoms of PMS. **Mustard** is indicated for depression which is also a common feature. **Cherry Plum** is the Remedy for suicidal tendencies and a fear of losing control. **Crab Apple** is valuable for those feelings of self-disgust and ugliness which often accompany the bloatedness, spots and blemishes which may occur. **Willow** will help feelings of self-pity which women can experience premenstrually. Finally **Hornbeam** is beneficial for fatigue and lethargy, encouraging an optimistic and enthusiastic outlook.

DIET

Since the increase in the number of PMS sufferers has risen partly due to the changes in dietary habits which have occurred, attention to diet is a crucial part of any PMS programme. Dr Guy Abraham, PMS pioneer, claims that 90 per cent of women will respond to a nutritional programme.

The following points are some of the dietary recommendations for PMS:

▶ *Reduce salt consumption which leads to fluid retention and weight gain.*
▶ *Reduce the consumption of refined sugar which leads to psychological symptoms.*
▶ *Reduce drinks which contain caffeine (coffee, tea, cola) and alcohol – these aggravate psychological symptoms.*
▶ *Reduce fats and protein.*
▶ *Increase your fibre intake by eating plenty of green, leafy vegetables, fruits and legumes to aid the elimination of toxins.*

Supplements which PMS sufferers have found to be useful include evening primrose oil, B vitamins (especially B_6), and vitamins C, D, E, calcium (1200 mg daily) and magnesium (alleviates irritability, fatigue, depression and oedema).

Fish oils and flax seed oils are good, but blackcurrant and borage oil could be better as many PMS sufferers are unable to convert linoleic acid and gamma linoleic acid and borage and blackcurrant seed oils are pre-formed GLA. It is also essential to reduce stress – aromatherapy, of course, is a wonderful way to relax. Gentle exercise such as yoga, swimming or walking can also decrease tension, improve circulation and prevent fluid retention.

Oils for other problems

The following essential oils may be applied, using any of the methods outlined in Chapter 3. Sitz baths, compresses and gentle massage of the abdomen and low back are particularly recommended for the treatment of women's problems.

Cystitis
Angelica seed, bergamot, cajeput, carrot seed, cedarwood, chamomile, cypress, eucalyptus, frankincense, geranium, juniper, lavender, lemon, myrtle, niaouli, palmarosa, pine, sandalwood, tea tree and thyme.

Herpes
Bergamot, eucalyptus, garlic, geranium, immortelle, lavender, lemon, melissa, niaouli and ravensara.

Infertility
Angelica seed, basil, carrot seed, clary sage, geranium, jasmine, melissa and rose.

Leucorrhea (white/yellow vaginal discharge)
Benzoin, bergamot, cedarwood, cinnamon, eucalyptus, geranium, hyssop, juniper, lavender, myrrh, myrtle, niaouli, rose, rosemary, sandalwood, tea tree and thyme.

Thrush (candida)
Bergamot, eucalyptus, frankincense, lavender, lemon, myrrh, patchouli, rosemary, rosewood, tea tree and thyme.

Vaginitis (vaginal inflammation)
German/Roman chamomile, clary sage, lavender, sandalwood, tea tree and thyme.

TEST YOUR KNOWLEDGE

1 If you were making a compress to relieve menstrual pain which two of the following oils would be particularly effective?
Carrot seed, lavender, neroli, peppermint

2 Which two of the following oils could help to relieve hot flushes experienced during the menopause?
Bergamot, black pepper, cypress, peppermint

3 Which Bach Flower Remedy helps a woman to cope with the change of the menopause?

4 Which oil can be used to reduce the cravings for sweet things which is characteristic of PMS?

5 To combat anger, irritability and balance mood swings associated with PMS which two of the following oils could be used?
Chamomile, fennel, geranium, rosemary

6 Which Bach Flower Remedy is indicated for irritability and impatience?

14

Pregnancy, childbirth, babies and children

In this chapter you will learn:
- *how aromatherapy may be used to treat a wide range of conditions throughout pregnancy safely and effectively*
- *how essential oils can help new mothers during and after childbirth*
- *how babies and children can benefit from aromatherapy*
- *which Bach Flower Remedies to take*
- *the importance of diet in pregnancy and for children.*

Aromatherapy may be used successfully throughout the 40 weeks of pregnancy to treat a wide range of conditions. Although no one can guarantee a healthy, normal baby, the risks can be substantially reduced if the mother takes good care of herself, follows a healthy diet and maintains a balanced state of mind (see pages 298–300 for Bach Flower Remedies and for an advised diet). There is a great deal of controversy about which oils to avoid in the various stages of pregnancy, particularly during the first trimester. Provided essential oils are used correctly and in the appropriate dilutions, there is no risk. In my own practice I have been privileged to treat many pregnant women with excellent results and no harmful side-effects. Indeed on both occasions when I was pregnant I was fortunate to be able to practise aromatherapy until the deliveries. Every week, on average, I was probably using about 20–30 different blends of essential oils on my clients. Both my pregnancies were problem-free with easy births without orthodox analgesia and two extremely healthy babies. I am certain that I could not have achieved this without my precious essential oils.

Although you should be aware of the potential hazards of some essential oils, it is vital to keep it all in perspective. Instead of giving you a long list of so-called hazardous oils – some of which are referred to with no proof – I recommend that you use the oils which I have indicated for each condition. Naturally if symptoms are severe or persist then the advice of a doctor should always be sought.

Common ailments in pregnancy

BACKACHE

Backache can become so severe that the mother can be incapacitated. Essential oils are marvellous for treating backache and they can be added to the bath, blended into a back rub or used in compresses.

Essential oils for backache: **German/Roman chamomile, black pepper, frankincense, geranium, ginger, lavender, marjoram and niaouli.**

Add six drops of any of the above oils to a warm bath and relax.

For a back massage the following combinations may be useful:

| 2 drops German/ Roman chamomile 1 drop geranium 1 drop lavender | or | 1 drop frankincense 1 drop ginger 1 drop rose | diluted in 10 ml of carrier oil |

Insight

A warm compress can be really useful for relieving backache associated with pregnancy. Try three drops chamomile and three drops lavender.

CONSTIPATION

It is vital for the pregnant woman to eat lots of 'natural' foods with plenty of fruit, vegetables and fibre. Also drink lots of water. Pregnancy is not the time to take chemical laxatives, which could be dangerous. Natural laxatives such as prunes are recommended and work excellently in combination with aromatherapy to ensure a regular bowel action.

Essential oils for constipation: **black pepper, German/Roman chamomile, lavender, lemon, patchouli, rose** and **marjoram.**

These oils may be used in a bath up to a maximum of six drops in total. The best method is to make up a massage blend and rub it into the abdomen in a clockwise direction (see *Get Started in Massage* for a full description of abdominal massage).

Aromatic formulae for constipation

1 drop black pepper
1 drop lavender
1 drop marjoram
} or
1 drop German/Roman chamomile
1 drop patchouli
1 drop rose
} diluted in 10 ml of carrier oil

CRAMP

Cramps in the legs appear to be more prevalent during the last months of the pregnancy and are often worse during the night. One possible cause may be a lack of calcium.

Essential oils for cramps: **German/Roman chamomile, cypress, frankincense, geranium, lavender, marjoram** and **rosemary.**

These oils may be used successfully in a footbath, or the legs can be gently massaged upwards from the ankle to the thigh.

Footbath for leg cramps
    2 drops cypress
    1 drop frankincense
    1 drop geranium
    2 drops lavender

Aromatic formulae for leg cramps

2 drops German/ Roman chamomile		2 drops German/ Roman chamomile	diluted
2 drops cypress	or	2 drops geranium	in 20 ml of carrier
2 drops lavender		2 drops marjoram	oil

FATIGUE

Extreme tiredness can be a problem in pregnancy, especially if the woman has other children to care for.

Essential oils for fatigue: **bergamot, geranium, grapefruit, lavender, lemon, lemongrass, lime, mandarin, neroli** and **rosemary**.

Insight

For a 'quick fix' burst of energy the best method is inhalation. Sprinkle a couple of drops of any of the above oils (the citrus oil lime is my particular favourite) on to a tissue and inhale deeply.

Add six drops of any of the recommended oils to a bath or footbath or treat yourself to a massage using one of the following blends:

2 drops bergamot		2 drops grapefruit	diluted in
2 drops geranium	or	2 drops lime	10 ml of
2 drops lemon		2 drops neroli	carrier oil

MORNING SICKNESS

Although nausea is commonly experienced during the early stages, some women are unlucky enough to be subject to it right through pregnancy.

Essential oils for nausea: **ginger, lavender, lemon, mandarin, melissa, peppermint, petitgrain** and **rosewood**.

Add any of the above oils to your morning bath. A particularly lovely combination is two drops of ginger, two drops of mandarin and two drops of petitgrain. A few sips of apple or orange juice prior to rising can prevent the excessive drop in blood sugar which accompanies nausea. A piece of dry toast or a biscuit before getting up can also be effective.

Insight

An excellent method of using essential oils for morning sickness is by inhalation. Simply sprinkle two to three drops of ginger, mandarin or peppermint on to a tissue, handkerchief or cotton wool ball and inhale deeply.

STRETCH MARKS

In order to prevent unsightly stretch marks, massage the abdomen twice daily in a clockwise direction. This has worked for me and all my clients. Massage of the abdomen is also a wonderful way to establish contact and form a strong bond with your baby.

Essential oils for preventing stretch marks: **carrot seed, German/ Roman chamomile, frankincense, geranium, lavender, lemon, mandarin, neroli** and **rose**.

Aromatic formula for stretch marks

1 drop carrot seed
2 drops frankincense
1 drop lavender
2 drops mandarin
2 drops neroli
1 drop rose

} diluted in 30 ml of carrier oil

Make up the above blend, shake well and store it in an amber-coloured glass bottle. Add a little wheatgerm oil to whichever carrier oil(s) you have selected.

Insight

As well as massaging the abdomen, you should also treat other areas which are susceptible to stretch marks – thighs, buttocks, breasts and upper chest.

VARICOSE VEINS

To prevent the arrival of varicose veins caused by the extra pressure on the legs, pregnant women should ideally rest with their legs raised for at least half an hour a day. If you can manage to raise them several times a day for five to ten minutes this will also help considerably.

Essential oils for varicose veins: **cypress, geranium, lavender, lemon** and **sandalwood**.

Gentle massage of the legs twice a day is also an excellent preventive treatment.

Aromatic formula for varicose veins

1 drop cypress ⎫
1 drop geranium ⎬ diluted in 10 ml of carrier oil
1 drop lemon ⎭

Footbaths are also quite effective. Try two drops each of cypress, geranium and lemon in a bowl of hand-hot water.

Bach Flower Remedies in pregnancy

During pregnancy women experience a variety of emotional ups and downs as well as the physical conditions described above. The Bach Flower Remedies are an excellent way of maintaining balance throughout the nine months of pregnancy. They are harmless and cause no side-effects.

Walnut is essential for coping with the enormous physical and emotional changes that take place so quickly in pregnancy. It is the must-have remedy for pregnancy.

Star of Bethlehem is for counteracting the shock – even when pregnancies are planned it still comes as a big shock when it actually happens. **Mimulus** is to alleviate the fears that the mother may be harbouring. Will the baby be normal? Can I cope with the pain? Will there be any complications? **Olive** is to combat fatigue and tiredness which is so often experienced. **Red Chestnut** is for overconcern for the baby's welfare (I have treated some pregnant women who have not wanted to have a bath in case it damages the baby). **Impatiens** is particularly useful towards the end of pregnancy when the end is in sight. Women understandably feel impatient and frustrated that the baby is not here, particularly when it is overdue. **Rescue Remedy** is ideal for the stages of labour when women can panic and lose control. If the mind is not relaxed then the contractions will be more painful. **Mustard** is the classic remedy for postnatal depression which descends out of the blue for no apparent reason. **Star of Bethlehem** should be taken if the birth was traumatic as well as **Walnut** to make the transition easier.

Diet in pregnancy

To give your baby the best possible start I recommend the following guidelines:

▶ *Eat plenty of fresh fruit and vegetables, especially dark green, leafy vegetables, wholegrains and an adequate amount of protein.*
▶ *Avoid refined carbohydrates (cakes, biscuits, sweets), processed foods, foods with artificial additives and excessive tea and coffee.*

- *Take a vitamin and mineral supplement and folic acid, if possible, prior to conception.*
- *Avoid excessive vitamin A which can cause congenital malformations. In the UK the Department of Health advises women not to eat liver due to its high vitamin A content.*
- *Avoid alcohol which has been associated with abnormalities.*
- *Stop smoking as this has been associated with a low birthweight.*
- *Avoid drugs. Check out all your medications whether prescribed by your doctor or bought over the counter.*
- *Avoid refined soft cheeses (e.g. camembert), pâté, uncooked eggs, mayonnaise (unless you use dairy-free, egg-free mayo), raw or uncooked meats and unpasteurized milk.*
- *Wash your hands after coming into contact with animals.*
- *Water! It has been theorized that morning sickness occurs when suboptimal quantities of water are consumed by the mother and the nausea that occurs during morning sickness may be a manifestation of thirst from the unborn foetus.*
- *Increase intake of the herb basil as it will improve the blood circulation.*
- *Increase intake of magnesium as it can help to alleviate muscle cramps.*
- *Maximize calcium intake as this is essential during pregnancy.*
- *Drinking plenty of juices and smoothies can be beneficial.*

Oils for other pregnancy problems

Haemorrhoids
Cypress, frankincense, geranium, lavender, lemon, myrrh and sandalwood. Best method: sitz bath/cream.

Heartburn
Bergamot, coriander, ginger, lemon, mandarin and sandalwood. Best method: massage of abdomen.

Hypertension (high blood pressure)
German/Roman chamomile, lavender, sandalwood and ylang ylang. Best method: inhalation/bath/massage.

Insomnia
German/Roman chamomile, lavender, mandarin, marjoram (sweet), neroli, sandalwood and ylang ylang. Best method: inhalation/bath/massage.

Mood swings/depression
Bergamot, cedarwood, clary sage, cypress, geranium, mandarin, neroli, rose and rosewood. Best method: inhalation/bath/massage.

Oedema
Cypress, geranium, lemon and mandarin. Best method: massage.

Urinary tract infections
Bergamot, German/Roman chamomile, cypress, juniper, sandalwood and tea tree. Best method: sitz bath.

Vaginal infections
Bergamot, lavender, myrrh and tea tree. Best method: sitz bath.

Childbirth

Essential oils are increasing in popularity with midwives, and some hospitals even have a stock of their own. Giving birth is extremely hard work but it is a wonderful, rewarding experience. Essential oils can stimulate the uterus to contract, facilitating the birth, and enable the mother to relax, thus affording pain relief.

ESSENTIAL OILS FOR LABOUR

Bergamot, clary sage, frankincense, geranium, jasmine, lavender, mandarin, marjoram, neroli, palmarosa, peppermint, petitgrain, rose otto and ylang ylang.

Aromatic formulae for labour

3 drops clary sage		3 drops frankincense	diluted
2 drops mandarin	or	2 drops lavender	in 30 ml
2 drops rose		2 drops neroli	of carrier
2 drops ylang ylang		2 drops palmarosa	oil

The oils may be massaged into the back with the mother in a side-lying position or on all fours (see *Get Started in Massage* for special techniques), or the mother's feet can be massaged.

> **Insight**
>
> For pain relief and relaxation essential oils may be inhaled on a tissue or cotton-wool ball as an alternative to gas and air. Compresses are also excellent for pain relief.

Postnatal care

Essential oils are highly effective after childbirth not only for physical problems but also to prevent or banish stress, anxiety and postnatal depression.

BREASTFEEDING

Breast milk is, of course, the best possible start for your baby, providing antibodies to disease and reducing the risk of allergies. However, it is not always easy to breastfeed. Essential oils can usually provide the answer.

To promote the milk supply
Fennel, clary sage, jasmine and **lemongrass** can all help to promote lactation – an old-fashioned remedy is to chew fennel seeds. Drink fennel tea daily and massage the breasts three times a day after feeding time (not the nipples). Massage almond oil or wheatgerm oil into the nipples to prevent cracking. Ensure that you wash the breasts prior to a feed. Do not use fennel oil excessively in cases of epilepsy.

Aromatic formula for increasing milk supply

3 drops fennel		diluted in
2 drops lemongrass	or	20 ml of
1 drop clary sage		carrier oil

I can assure you that essential oils can promote the milk supply. I breastfed my daughter until she was 15 months old and my son until he was two years old. If you have no desire to breastfeed or perhaps wish to give up, the following oils will help to stop lactation: **cypress, geranium, lavender** and **peppermint**.

Aromatic formula for decreasing milk supply

2 drops cypress		diluted in 20 ml of
3 drops peppermint		carrier oil

Peppermint and **geranium** compresses are also good.

....

Insight

Mastitis is a common, painful disorder of the breasts. A compress with two drops of German/Roman chamomile, one drop of geranium, one drop of lavender and one drop of peppermint will help to cool down the inflammation.

....

HEALING THE PERINEUM

The perineum can become badly damaged during the birth process, particularly if you have torn badly or have had a forceps delivery. Aromatherapy sitz baths can increase the rate of healing, decrease the pain and fight off any infections. Compresses are also highly recommended.

Aromatic sitz bath for the perineum

2 drops German/ Roman chamomile		2 drops cypress
2 drops lavender	or	1 drop frankincense
2 drops tea tree		1 drop myrrh
		2 drops tea tree

If you have been unfortunate enough to have a Caesarean section, baths and compresses with three drops of **lavender** and three drops of **tea tree** will help the healing process. Do not massage the scar until it has fully healed.

POSTNATAL DEPRESSION

Although a few women suffer no emotional imbalance at all, the majority suffer from the 'baby blues' a few days after the birth. There are many essential oils to strengthen the nervous system and uplift the despondency and despair.

Essential oils for the 'baby blues': **bergamot, clary sage, frankincense, geranium, grapefruit, jasmine, mandarin, melissa, neroli** and **rose.**

Choose one oil or a combination from the list above using a maximum of six drops in the bath. The new mother should also take some time out each week to indulge herself in an aromatherapy massage.

Aromatherapy for babies

Babies love essential oils, particularly if their mother has used them throughout her pregnancy, and they respond so rapidly to them. The use of essential oils helps to boost the immune system and if the body does become ill, the recovery will be much speedier and the baby will experience far less discomfort.

Massage is a powerful and wonderful way for the parents to bond with their baby – I have described a detailed massage routine in *Get Started in Massage.*

Essential oils are used in low dilutions for aromamassage and baths. Babies should never be given essential oils internally.

....

Insight

For babies up to the age of 12 months, the appropriate dilutions are:

Babies (0–2 months): 1 drop per 15 ml carrier oil in a massage; 1 drop in the bath.

Babies (2–12 months): 1 drop per 10 ml carrier oil in a massage; 1 drop in the bath.

....

COLIC

Colic is a distressing condition for both the baby and the parents. The baby continues to cry even when picked up, which makes the parents feel helpless. However, essential oils can provide an answer.

One drop of **German/Roman chamomile** or one drop of **mandarin** can be added to 15 ml of carrier oil and massaged gently into the baby's abdomen.

If the baby continues to cry, try a compress of **German/Roman chamomile**. Add one drop of German/Roman chamomile to a small amount of water in a bowl. Stir well and soak a flannel in the solution. Place the flannel on the baby's abdomen.

If the colic persists, the mother should consider her diet carefully. Perhaps the baby is allergic to the dairy foods that she is eating? It is also well worth the effort to take the baby to see a fully qualified osteopath who has experience in the cranial field with babies.

COUGHS AND COLDS

Aromatherapy is an excellent way of preventing babies from picking up coughs and colds. If someone in the household has a cold, the baby can be protected by using essential oils in a diffuser or by using the plant spray method (see page 29). **Tea tree, eucalyptus, cajeput, myrtle** and **niaouli** are all excellent oils to diffuse.

You may also place under the baby's cot a small bowl of boiling water to which you have added one drop of cajeput/myrtle and one drop of tea tree.

> **Insight**
> One drop of **lavender** and one drop of **myrtle** on a piece of cotton wool placed at the bottom of the crib or the cot will help the baby to breathe and sleep more easily.

CRADLE CAP

'Cradle cap' is the term given to 'crusting' on the scalp. It is easy to relieve with essential oils. My favourite oil for this is **geranium**. Add one drop of geranium to 15 ml of sweet almond oil and massage gently into the scalp. This mixture should be used daily until the cradle cap subsides.

INSOMNIA/RESTLESSNESS

It is often difficult to get a baby into a sleeping routine which suits the parents. Some babies like to sleep in the day and wake up in the night. To establish a good pattern put one drop of **lavender** and one drop of **German/Roman chamomile** into a diffuser or vaporizer and light it or switch it on about half an hour before bedtime, ensuring that you close the bedroom door.

Alternatively, under the cot place a small bowl of boiling water to which you have added two drops of German/Roman chamomile.

NAPPY RASH

Nappy rash can be prevented and treated by essential oils. When you change the baby, avoid using chemically perfumed 'baby wipes'. Instead add one drop of **German/Roman chamomile** or **lavender** or **yarrow** to one pint of water and agitate the water thoroughly. With my two children I used to put a drop in the sink and dip them in to clean their bottoms. You can also add essential oils to a jar of pure organic skin cream or zinc and castor oil cream.

Add approximately one drop per 15 g. To a 60 g jar of cream, add two drops of German/Roman chamomile, one drop of lavender and one drop of yarrow. To a 100 g jar, add two drops of German/Roman chamomile, two drops of lavender and two drops of yarrow.

TEETHING

Teething usually begins around four to six months although there are wide variations and it has been known for a baby to be born with teeth. Teething can be a painful experience for the baby and for the parents who often have to endure many sleepless nights. **German/Roman chamomile**, **lavender** and **yarrow** are three of the best essential oils for teething.

Insight

My favourite method for teething is to put one drop of Roman Chamomile into an egg cup full of carrier oil. Stir the mixture well and using your finger or a cotton bud, massage baby's gums and also massage externally on the affected side of the face.

Bach Flower Remedies for babies

The Bach Flower Remedies can be of enormous help to babies who usually respond much more rapidly to them than adults. They have not yet accumulated all the 'emotional baggage' which some adults carry around with them and the Remedies can get to work straightaway.

Insight

Star of Bethlehem 'for shock' should always be administered after the birth, especially if it was a traumatic birth. Birth is a difficult enough journey even without any complications. If the mother is breastfeeding she can take the remedy and it will be imparted through the breast milk. Otherwise add the remedy to the baby's bottle.

Olive is an essential remedy for the parents since it is indicated for weariness and exhaustion – I have never met parents who are not tired! The whole family should take **Walnut** to help them to adjust to the idea of a new baby in the house. **Chicory** is for sleepy, drowsy babies who are clingy and do not want to be left on their own. **Clematis** is for sleepy, drowsy babies who do not even bother to wake up for feeds. These babies have a 'far away' look in their eyes and appear to have no interest in this world. **Mimulus** can be prescribed for fearful, nervous babies who are easily startled and usually cry on awakening. **Vervain** can help overactive babies who seem unable to relax and have great difficulty in going to sleep.

Aromatherapy for children

Children also respond very rapidly to the effects of essential oils. Their innate powers of self-healing enable them to throw off toxins very quickly because their bodies are not impaired by years of bad diet, lack of exercise, negative thoughts, pollution and stress.

Essential oils should never be given internally to young children. You should not try to treat serious illnesses or indeed any illnesses which have not been diagnosed by a qualified medical practitioner.

Insight

Suitable dilutions for children are:

Small children (1–5 years): 1–2 drops per 10 ml carrier oil in a massage; 2 drops in the bath (add to a teaspoon of carrier oil).

Juniors (5–12 years): 2–3 drops per 10 ml carrier oil in a massage; 3–4 drops in the bath (add to a teaspoon of carrier oil).

Adolescents (12 years +): 3 drops per 10 ml carrier oil in a massage; 4–5 drops in the bath.

ALLERGIES (E.G. ECZEMA)

Food allergies are very common in children and are responsible for many hyperactivity and behavioural problems. Children may be sensitive to additives and preservatives, as well as dairy foods, sugar and wheat.

German/Roman chamomile, lavender or **yarrow** can be added to the bath water in the appropriate dilution. These oils may also be added to a pure organic skin cream or moisturizing lotion and applied several times daily, depending upon the severity of the condition, to ease discomfort, inflammation and itching. Essential oils such as **geranium, melissa, neroli, rose** and **sandalwood** will help if the allergy is stress-related, and should be added to the daily bath.

If possible the food(s) or other offending substances causing the reaction(s) should be isolated and eliminated.

ASTHMA

Asthma attacks are very frightening for young children and their parents. They can be related to allergies to food and environmental factors such as house dust. Stress will increase the severity and frequency of the attacks.

Aromatherapy treatment is aimed at reducing the anxiety and improving the function of the lungs. Essential oils useful for asthma include: **cypress, frankincense, lavender, marjoram, melissa, neroli, German/Roman chamomile** and **rose**. A blend of any of these oils can be massaged into the upper back and chest. Alternatively, put one drop of essential oil on a handkerchief or tissue and inhale deeply.

Asthma formulae
CHILD (1–5 YEARS)

1 drop lavender 1 drop German/ Roman chamomile	} or	1 drop German/ Roman chamomile 1 drop neroli	} diluted in 10 ml of carrier oil

CHILD (5–12 YEARS)

1 drop frankincense		1 drop cypress		diluted in
1 drop lavender	or	1 drop frankincense		10 ml of
1 drop marjoram		1 drop German/		carrier oil
		Roman chamomile		

ATHLETE'S FOOT (TINEA PEDIS)

This fungal infection found in between the toes is often picked up by children at swimming pools and in changing rooms. The skin becomes damp, flaky, itchy, spongy and white.

Useful essential oils include: **cypress, lavender, lemon** and **tea tree.** The child should be encouraged to have at least two footbaths daily, to which you have added one, or a combination, of the oils suggested above. One drop of lavender and one drop of tea tree is an excellent combination. These essential oils may also be added to two teaspoons of carrier oil dabbed in between the toes.

The skin should be kept as dry as possible between the toes and only cotton or wool socks should be worn (not nylon or synthetic fibres).

BRUISES

Immediately after a bump, essential oils may be applied on an ice-cold compress. Add one drop of **lavender** and one drop of **German/Roman chamomile** to a small bowl of cold water. Use a flannel to soak up the solution, wring it out and apply to the affected area.

BURNS

Hold the affected area under running cold water then apply a cold compress to which you have added two drops of pure essential oil of **lavender**. Other useful oils for burns include **German/Roman chamomile** and **yarrow**.

COUGHS AND COLDS

The antibacterial and antiviral properties of essential oils are extremely effective when treating coughs and colds.

If the child has a fever then **lavender, German/Roman chamomile** and **tea tree** are beneficial. Place one drop of each into a small bowl of lukewarm water and sponge down the body and head until the fever subsides. Alternatively, make a cold compress to which you have added these oils, and place it on the back of the neck or forehead or wrap it around the feet.

For coughs, massage the chest, throat and upper back using a blend containing the appropriate number of drops of essential oils chosen from: **cajeput, cypress, eucalyptus, frankincense, lavender, myrtle, German/Roman chamomile, rosemary** or **tea tree**. These oils will help to fight the infection, expel the mucus, relieve bronchial spasm and induce relaxation.

Coughs and colds formulae
CHILD (1–5 YEARS)

1 drop lavender	1 drop lavender	diluted in 10 ml of
1 drop tea tree	1 drop myrtle	carrier oil

CHILD (5–12 YEARS)

1 drop cajeput	1 drop frankincense	diluted in
1 drop lavender	1 drop myrtle	10 ml of
1 drop tea tree	1 drop German/	carrier oil
	Roman chamomile	

CUTS AND GRAZES

It is very important to clean the area thoroughly to prevent any infection. Useful essential oils include **lavender, lemon** and **tea tree**. Bathe the wound with warm water to which you have added one drop of lavender plus one drop of tea tree. This will calm the child and will not sting as much as a proprietary antiseptic.

> **Insight**
> If a dressing is needed on a cut or a graze, one drop of neat lavender on a sticking plaster will accelerate the healing process.

DIGESTIVE PROBLEMS

Constipation in children can be caused by poor eating habits or even by stress. Encourage your children to eat plenty of fresh fruit and vegetables in preference to 'junk food' and to drink plenty of water and fruit juices to reduce dehydration of the stools. Straining should be avoided; do not put your children under pressure to 'perform' on the toilet.

Useful essential oils to treat constipation include: **geranium, mandarin, marjoram, German/Roman chamomile** and **rosemary**. The best method of application is to massage the abdomen daily, working in a clockwise direction.

Constipation formulae

CHILD (1–5 YEARS)		CHILD (5–12 YEARS)	
1 drop mandarin 1 drop German/Roman chamomile	} or	2 drops mandarin 1 drop marjoram	} diluted in 10 ml of carrier oil

Diarrhoea may be caused by an infection, an allergy to food, certain drugs or by stress. It is vital to replace lost fluid to prevent dehydration. Avoid food but drink as much liquid as possible. If the diarrhoea persists then consult a medically qualified practitioner.

Useful essential oils for diarrhoea include: **geranium, ginger, lavender, neroli, German/Roman chamomile** and **sandalwood**. A massage blend may be gently rubbed into the abdomen and compresses may be applied to help to alleviate pain.

Diarrhoea formulae

CHILD (1–5 YEARS)	CHILD (5–12 YEARS)	
1 drop lavender	1 drop ginger	diluted in
1 drop neroli	1 drop neroli	10 ml of
	or 1 drop German/	carrier oil
	Roman chamomile	

EARACHE

Blend one drop of either **lavender** or **German/Roman chamomile** with a teaspoon of olive oil. Soak a piece of cotton wool in this mixture and place it in the ear. If pain is severe, rub any swollen glands, using the appropriate number of drops of **lavender** and **German/Roman chamomile**. If the earache is recurrent, visit an osteopath who specializes in children.

HEAD LICE

Please refer to page 269.

Diet tips for children

▶ *Veggie sticks – when stacked into a fast food restaurant chip holder, they look like chips, but they're so much healthier! Variety is vital, so give them sticks of peppers, carrots, celery and so on.*

▶ *Sandwiches – if you make sandwiches, brown bread is best, but make sure to add some veggies too, such as cucumber, cress or coleslaw. Make sure you offer a variety of fillings, such as tuna, egg, ham, hummus, cheese, salad, chicken, etc. Try cutting the bread into shapes, or roll up tortilla flat breads.*

▶ *Healthy crisps – the problem with most crisps is that they are fattening and are cooked in hydrogenated vegetable oil (linked to cancer). Healthier options now available are banana chips, fruit leathers or pure apple crisps.*

- Cereal bars and flapjacks – like crisps, many are fattening and contain hydrogenated vegetable oil, so you might need to visit a health food shop. Home-made ones are best!
- Fruit – again, choose a different fruit daily and try some combinations with fruit kebabs. Fruit smoothies are a winning after-school treat. For special occasions try a fondue with melted organic chocolate and a fruit platter.
- Variety is the spice of life! With the multitude of different biochemical processes going on inside each and every one of us every day, it is essential that we get a wide variety of vitamins and minerals. The best way to get these is by eating a range of different fruit and vegetables.
- Dazzle your kids with colour! Kids love colour, so use this to their advantage by getting them to eat a multi-coloured fruit or a vegetable snack every day.
- Water – absolutely vital! With a little freshly squeezed juice it tastes nice, too. Avoid fizzy drinks and sweetened juices. Remember, your little sweethearts should be 70 per cent water, not pop!
- Make a weekly planner – get your children to plan their week's healthy snacks. Then go to the supermarket and see if they can find the ingredients. Remember to be creative and make it fun. Learn together how to sprout seeds and make vegetable juices in a juicer. Try blueberry muffins, individual pizzas, tacos with ten different fillings so they can create their own, oatmeal cookies with flax seeds hidden in them. If you're enthusiastic, they will be too!
- Friday is treat day – if your kids can't live without their chocolate bar or fizzy drink (they can really!) tell them they can have them on Friday (but only if they've behaved themselves during the week!). It may seem tough but you know more about nutrition than they do.

INFECTIOUS DISEASES

Chickenpox
Add **lavender** and **German/Roman chamomile** to the bath.
Add either German/Roman chamomile and lavender, or

German/Roman chamomile and tea tree, to moisturizing lotion and massage.

Measles
Use **German/Roman chamomile** and **lavender** in oil or moisturizing lotion and massage gently.

Mumps
Blend the appropriate number of drops into a massage oil using **lavender, lemon** or **tea tree.**

Rubella (German measles)
Blend the appropriate number of drops into a massage oil using **lavender, German/Roman chamomile** or **tea tree.**

Whooping cough
Blend the appropriate number of drops for the child's age into a massage oil and rub the chest and add one drop to the child's pillow using **cypress, lavender, myrtle, rosemary** or **tea tree.**

TEST YOUR KNOWLEDGE

1 *Choose two oils which can combat morning sickness.*
   Ginger, frankincense, mandarin, patchouli

2 *How would you use the oils for morning sickness?*

3 *Choose three oils which can help to prevent stretchmarks.*
   Bergamot, frankincense, lemon, neroli, niaouli, peppermint,
   rose

4 *Which of the following combinations of oils would be suitable*
   for childbirth?
   a *myrrh/rosewood/tea tree*
   b *clary sage/lavender/rose*

5 *Which method of use is particularly suitable for treating*
   mastitis?

6 *How many drops of essential oil would you use in a bath for a*
   baby up to the age of 12 months?

7 *Which oil is useful for colic?*
   a *chamomile*
   b *tea tree*

8 *How many drops of essential oil would you use in the bath for*
   a child aged 1–5?

9 *Choose two oils suitable for treating a child's cough.*
   Lavender, myrtle, peppermint, rose

10 *Would lavender or mandarin help to heal a cut?*

15

Sensual aromatherapy
for couples

In this chapter you will learn:

- *how aromatherapy can make you more sexually attractive*
- *how to enhance your love life*
- *how aromatherapy may help you to overcome sexual difficulties*
- *which Bach Flower Remedies to take.*

All of us have our own natural body scent and we can be attracted to another person by the way that he or she smells. Aromas can have erotic connotations. Sexual arousal causes the body to release all sorts of exotic odours – especially from the skin, breath and sexual organs. It is possible to enhance these odours by using essential oils to make ourselves more sexually attractive.

There are many ways of using essential oils to enhance your love life and to achieve sexual fulfilment.

Insight

The aroma of a 'love potion' must of course suit *both* your tastes. Aroma preference is important when deciding which essential oils to blend together, as we are instinctively drawn to those essential oils which we need.

Scenting

It is easy to perfume your own lingerie. When you are washing
your delicate and seductive items by hand, just add two drops of
essential oil to the final rinse. If you are washing by machine then
put four drops to a small amount of water and add to the final
rinse in the softener section.

Sensual oils for your lingerie
Bergamot, geranium, neroli and **ylang ylang** are all excellent
choices. It is advisable not to use absolutes or the thick heavy oils
to perfume your lingerie as they may stain the fabric.

You can also perfume your lingerie in your chest of
drawers and in your wardrobe. Sprinkle about six drops of
essential oils of **rose, myrtle, jasmine, neroli, bergamot,
geranium, ylang ylang, patchouli, frankincense** or **sandalwood,**
or whatever your preference is, on to cotton-wool balls and
place them in greaseproof bags. Prick holes in the bags to allow
the wonderful fragrances to permeate into your clothing.
Place these bags into your drawers or hang them up inside your
wardrobe.

Beautiful aromatic silk bags make wonderful presents.
Cut out a circle of silk and stitch around the circumference with
a thick thread. Place a cotton-wool ball which has been sprinkled
with essential oils into the centre of the silk circle. Gather up the
thread so that the cotton-wool ball(s) is enclosed by the silk. Sew
on a piece of thin ribbon so that you can hang up your pomander.
Particularly suitable essential oils would be: **frankincense, patchouli,
rose, jasmine, vetivert** and **ylang ylang,** as these aromas will last a
long time.

Insight

It is easy to make your own drawer liners to perfume your clothes. Sprinkle six drops of essential oil on to squares of blotting paper or any absorbent pieces of paper.

SCENTING YOUR BEDLINEN

Scented bedlinen is sensual and it is easy to do. There are several methods:

▶ *Put four drops of essential oil into a small amount of water and add to the softener section of your washing machine for the final rinse.*

▶ *Fill a small plant spray with spring water, add ten drops of the essential oils of your own choice and then spray the bottom sheet lightly.*

▶ *Put a few drops of your chosen essential oils on to cotton-wool balls or on to pieces of absorbent, natural material and place them between the sheets in your airing cupboard, or inside your pillow case.*

SCENTING YOUR BEDROOM

A clay burner or radiator fragrancer is the perfect way to create a romantic and sensual environment. Put a few teaspoons of water into the loose bowl on top of your clay burner and sprinkle six drops into it. Light the night light to allow the oils to diffuse into the air.

Suggested recipes for your burner

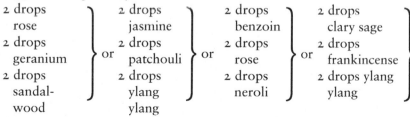

2 drops rose
2 drops geranium
2 drops sandal-wood

or

2 drops jasmine
2 drops patchouli
2 drops ylang ylang

or

2 drops benzoin
2 drops rose
2 drops neroli

or

2 drops clary sage
2 drops frankincense
2 drops ylang ylang

For a more masculine aroma

3 drops cedar wood 3 drops sandal-wood	or	2 drops black pepper 2 drops ylang ylang 2 drops lemon/mandarin	or	3 drops benzoin 3 drops sandal-wood	or	2 drops bergamot 2 drops ginger 2 drops vetivert

> **Insight**
>
> Women particularly love jasmine, rose, neroli and ylang ylang. Men particularly love cedarwood, sandalwood, vetivert and ylang ylang.

Candles are also perfect for scenting your bedroom and creating a romantic scene. Light your candle and wait until the wax has slightly melted and then carefully put one to two drops of essential oil into the melted wax, taking care to avoid the wick.

> **Insight**
>
> ▶ *To a pink candle add essential oil of rose to encourage new love, romance and gentleness.*
> ▶ *To a red candle add ylang ylang to induce passion and sexuality.*
> ▶ *To a violet candle add frankincense to add an air of mystery.*

Massage

Massage is an excellent way of arousing your partner and it is not necessary to have had a training in massage to achieve the desired effect. Just follow your instincts. Pay particular attention to the abdominal area, especially the area from the navel to the pubis and the low back and buttocks. There are some effective points for boosting sexual energy and heightening sexual response.

To set the scene, scent your room with one of the recipes already suggested and light a few candles around the room. Refer to Chapter 7 in this book and my other book in this series *Get Started in Massage* for specific massage techniques.

The following essential oils are ideal for increasing sexual desire: **benzoin, bergamot, black pepper, cinnamon, clary sage, frankincense, ginger, jasmine, melissa, myrtle, neroli, palmarosa, patchouli, petitgrain, rose, sandalwood, vetivert** and **ylang ylang**.

Suggested massage blends

For women:		For men:	
2 drops jasmine		2 drops clary sage	diluted in
2 drops rose	or	2 drops ginger or	30 ml of
3 drops sandalwood		black pepper	carrier oil
2 drops ylang ylang		3 drops sandalwood	
		2 drops ylang ylang	

Sexual difficulties

VAGINAL DRYNESS

Lack of vaginal secretion can make intercourse difficult, uncomfortable or even impossible. Some of the factors affecting secretion include hormone imbalance, such as experienced at the menopause, the contraceptive pill or negative emotions.

A simple solution to this problem is to apply a small amount of jojoba to the vagina. However, this is only a temporary remedy. For the long term, essential oils which increase vaginal secretions (especially those that imitate the hormone oestrogen) should be used in the bath (six drops) or in massage blends (three to four drops to 10 ml of carrier oil).

Take a daily bath with one of the formulae and use the massage recipe every day for a week and you should notice an increase in secretion.

Bath formulae to overcome vaginal dryness

2 drops clary sage		2 drops fennel		1 drop melissa	
1 drop geranium	or	2 drops geranium	or	2 drops neroli	
3 drops rose		2 drops lavender		3 drops sandalwood	

Alternatively, use any of the oils mentioned in the formula singularly.

Massage formula
2 drops clary sage
2 drops fennel
2 drops rose
2 drops sandalwood

} diluted in 30 ml of carrier oil

IMPOTENCE

A temporary state of impotence can happen to any man.
The cause may be physical or emotional exhaustion, nervous tension, lack of confidence or a symptom of illness. Some drugs can affect the libido, for example valium and librium. Whatever the reason the following essential oils are invaluable. Choose any three, or use one of my suggested recipes: **basil, black pepper, cardamom, clary sage, coriander, cinnamon, geranium, ginger, jasmine, lavender, patchouli, rose, rosemary, rosewood, sandalwood, thyme, ylang ylang.**

Massage formulae for impotence

1 drop cinnamon 1 drop coriander 2 drops ginger 1 drop rosemary }	or	1 drop clary sage 2 drops ginger 1 drop jasmine 2 drops sandalwood }	or	2 drops black pepper 2 drops ginger 2 drops rosewood }	diluted in 20 ml of carrier oil }

Insight

For loss of libido as you massage your partner pay particular attention to the lower back, the abdominal area and upper thighs. Make sure that you avoid the genitals. Apply the oils for approximately ten days.

For men who suffer with premature ejaculation the following blend should be effective:

1 drop benzoin
2 drops marjoram   } diluted in 30 ml of carrier oil
1 drop vetivert

Bach Flower Remedies

The word 'impotence' has an enormous stigma attached to it and can put a strain on a marriage or partnership, resulting in endless rows or even eventually a rift in a relationship. Since impotence is often of emotional origin the Bach Flower Remedies are highly advantageous.

Larch is a wonderful Remedy for boosting a lack of confidence and feelings of inadequacy; **White Chestnut** is useful for the worries which a man has concerning his virility; **Olive** is essential for exhaustion whether physical or emotional; **Mimulus** is excellent for fear of failure.

FRIGIDITY

There are many factors which contribute to a lack of sexual response. The hormone which is responsible for the sex drive in both men and women is testosterone. Levels of testosterone vary not only between males and females but also among women. Those with high testosterone levels have a strong sexual appetite. Anxiety, or fear, perhaps from some traumatic experience in the past, can actually cause levels of this hormone to deplete. Fatigue and stress due to pressures with work, money or family will also lower the sex drive.

Boredom and lack of sexual satisfaction can also result in frigidity. Some women have never experienced an orgasm. If a man takes his partner for granted and does not indulge in any foreplay then this will eventually lead to sexual unresponsiveness or even aversion. Lack of libido may also be caused by stress and exhaustion. If a woman is working and has several children to look after it is little wonder if she loses her sex drive.

Essential oils to combat frigidity: **clary sage, ginger, jasmine, neroli, rose, sandalwood** and **ylang ylang** are all effective. Any of these oils can be used in your daily bath to stimulate and renew your interest in sex.

Massage formulae for frigidity

3 drops clary sage		3 drops ginger		diluted in
3 drops jasmine	or	3 drops rose		30 ml of
3 drops ylang ylang		3 drops ylang ylang		carrier oil

Use one of the recipes above for about ten days. The oils should be applied particularly to the upper thighs, abdomen and lower back.

Bach Flower Remedies
For the majority of women frigidity is of an emotional origin and the Bach Flower Remedies can be helpful. If the problem arises from exhaustion then **Olive** is the recommended Remedy.

For fear of sex **Mimulus** can help to ease the problem. **Honeysuckle** is beneficial where the woman has suffered a traumatic experience in the past such as rape. If this has led to a sense of being 'dirty' and 'contaminated', then **Crab Apple** would be beneficial. **Wild Rose** is helpful for those who suffer from boredom and have a submissive approach. **Willow** is valuable for the anger and resentment which the woman may experience if her partner is unable to satisfy her needs.

TEST YOUR KNOWLEDGE

1 When washing your lingerie by hand how many drops of essential oil would you add to the final rinse to perfume it?

2 How can you make your own drawer liners?

3 Choose two oils particularly suitable for sexual arousal in a woman.

  Black pepper, jasmine, rose, vetivert

4 To treat impotence which of the following would you use?
  a   fennel/grapefruit/lemon
  b   black pepper/ginger/jasmine

5 Which Bach Flower Remedy can boost confidence?

16

Where to go from here

In this chapter you will learn:
- *how to select a suitable aromatherapy college*
- *what to expect from a professional aromatherapy consultation.*

Professional training

If you have been inspired by this book you may want to take an aromatherapy course. There are many short and weekend courses available which will give you the skills to help your friends and relations with simple problems. Please check any course you go on is run by a fully qualified aromatherapist (unfortunately many are not). Any weekend or short course will not, however, enable you to practise professionally on the general public. A fully qualified aromatherapist will have studied for anything from nine months to two years part-time and will have a sound knowledge of anatomy, physiology, business studies and professional conduct as well as of massage and essential oils. Training also involves the completion of at least ten comprehensive case histories which have included over 60 treatments. As a registered practitioner, you will be required to undertake an amount of Continuing Professional Development (CPD) training to update your skills.

You should check that the aromatherapy establishment you choose is accredited to a reputable aromatherapy association.

The principal of the school should be a qualified teacher, preferably recognized by the Department of Education and Science, and should have at least five years' clinical aromatherapy experience.

You should also check that on completion of your course you will be adequately insured to practise aromatherapy. Some schools issue a certificate which is a worthless, and sometimes very expensive, piece of paper.

> **Insight**
> The best way to choose an aromatherapy college is by recommendation. If you are at all unsure, ask if you can visit the school or college to look round, and perhaps see some of the former students' coursework and case histories. Do not expect to receive identical aromatherapy training from every school. Some schools will offer topics in addition to the minimum requirements.

An aromatherapy consultation

If, after reading this book, you wish to try some aromatherapy treatments for yourself it is important to find a trained therapist so that you are not disappointed. The best way of finding a good aromatherapist is, again, by recommendation. You may well have to wait a while for the initial consultation – but this is a good sign!

Do not be afraid to ask questions when you telephone to book your consultation. Ask if the therapist belongs to a professional association and check that he/she is properly insured.

The initial consultation can take up to one-and-a-half hours, although a very experienced practitioner will probably need less time. The first 30 minutes will be taken up by a series of detailed questions which are necessary if the therapist is to make an accurate evaluation of the patient. A skilled therapist will try to find out the cause of your problems rather than merely treating your symptoms. After the aromatherapist has made the initial assessment the essential oils will be selected. The blend which is chosen must match the individual's needs in order to benefit him/her holistically. All aspects of you as a person are considered – physical, emotional and spiritual.

The aromatherapy massage consists of a variety of techniques, once again tailored to your individual needs. A 'standard' form of aromatherapy massage, in my view, is unacceptable – how can the same aromatherapy treatment be suitable for everyone?

At the end of the treatment, you should experience a sense of deep relaxation. It is possible, although not inevitable, that you will have some reactions as a result of the aromatherapy treatment, due to the release of toxins. Any reaction should be viewed as positive and desirable, since this is indicative of your body's innate capacity for self-healing and shows that the essential oils are working.

The frequency of your bowel movements may increase, and your stools may also build up in bulk and volume. This is excellent as it is an indication that your body is casting aside its rubbish. It may be necessary to urinate more frequently after a treatment, especially if you have been suffering from fluid retention. You might develop a cold, particularly if your nasal passages and the bronchial tubes need unblocking. You may even experience emotional changes or develop more positive changes in your attitude to life. But do not worry – you will not experience all of these reactions at once and any that you do will be only temporary. However, you may not experience any reactions at all. Most clients feel marvellous after a treatment and report an improved sense of well-being and an increase in vitality. Their only complaint is that after one treatment they are thoroughly addicted to aromatherapy!

You may be given advice to carry out at home. The aromatherapist may give you a massage blend or some essential oils to add to your daily bath. You may also be given dietary advice.

All in all, an aromatherapy treatment should be a highly pleasurable experience. I have tried a wide range of complementary therapies and I am totally committed to my monthly aromatherapy treatments, which I find beneficial. Enjoy your aromatherapy and let it become part of your everyday life!

Aromatherapy for common ailments: a therapeutic index

Circulatory/immune systems

Aids angelica seed, chamomiles, lavender, lemon, niaouli, tea tree, thyme

Anaemia black pepper, carrot seed, chamomiles, geranium, lemon, lime, peppermint, rosemary, thyme

Arteriosclerosis black pepper, cedarwood, ginger, juniper, lemon, rosemary, yarrow

Chilblains black pepper, ginger, lemon, marjoram

Fever angelica seed, black pepper, chamomiles, eucalyptus, ginger, juniper, lavender, peppermint

Glandular fever angelica seed, cypress, lavender, lemon, ravensara, tea tree, thyme

Haemorrhoids cypress, geranium, juniper, lemon, myrrh, yarrow

Heart *False angina*: neroli; *Irregular heartbeat* (tachycardia): marjoram, melissa, petitgrain, sandalwood, ylang ylang; *Tonic*: angelica seed, benzoin, lavender, marjoram, melissa, neroli, rose, sandalwood

High blood pressure chamomile, clary sage, lavender, lemon, marjoram, melissa, neroli, yarrow, ylang ylang

High cholesterol cedarwood, ginger, juniper, lemon, rosemary, thyme

Immune system booster cardamom, carrot seed, chamomiles, cinnamon, lavender, lemon, lemongrass, lime, mandarin, myrtle, niaouli, petitgrain, ravensara, tea tree, thyme, vetivert

Low blood pressure rosemary, thyme

Lymphatic congestion carrot seed, cedarwood, cypress, fennel, grapefruit, juniper, lemon, lime, mandarin, pine, rosemary

ME (myalgic encephalomyelitis) angelica seed, cypress, grapefruit, lavender, lemongrass, pine, ravensara, rosemary, rosewood, tea tree, thyme

Palpitations chamomiles, clary sage, lavender, melissa, neroli, petitgrain, rose, rosemary, ylang ylang

Poor circulation angelica seed, benzoin, black pepper, cardamom, carrot seed, cedarwood, cinnamon, coriander, cypress, eucalyptus, ginger, hyssop, lemon, lemongrass, lime, mandarin, marjoram, niaouli, pine, rosemary, thyme

Varicose veins cypress, geranium, ginger, lemon, neroli, tea tree, yarrow

---

Digestive system

Anorexia angelica seed, bergamot, black pepper, carrot seed, coriander, fennel, frankincense, jasmine, lavender, neroli, palmarosa, rose, thyme

Appetite balancer fennel, patchouli

Bulimia bergamot, clary sage, geranium, jasmine, lavender, neroli, rose

Candida chamomiles, cinnamon, citronella, ginger, myrrh, patchouli, rosemary, tea tree, thyme, yarrow

Colic bergamot, black pepper, chamomiles, clary sage, coriander, fennel, ginger, juniper, lavender, lemongrass, marjoram, peppermint, rosemary, yarrow

Colitis bergamot, black pepper, chamomiles, ginger, lavender, lemongrass, neroli, peppermint, rosemary, yarrow

Constipation black pepper, cardamom, carrot seed, cinnamon, fennel, ginger, hyssop, marjoram, patchouli, rose, rosemary, thyme

Diabetes eucalyptus, geranium, juniper

Diarrhoea black pepper, cajeput, chamomiles, cinnamon, coriander, cypress, eucalyptus, geranium, ginger, lavender, lemon, mandarin, myrrh, myrtle, neroli (*stress induced*), patchouli, petitgrain, peppermint, rosemary, sandalwood

Fistula (anal) geranium, lavender, lemon, tea tree

Flatulence angelica seed, basil, bergamot, black pepper, cardamom, carrot seed, chamomiles, coriander, fennel, ginger, hyssop, juniper, lavender, lemon, lemongrass, mandarin, marjoram, myrrh, neroli, peppermint, rosemary, thyme

Food poisoning black pepper, fennel, grapefruit, juniper, rosemary

Gall bladder bergamot, chamomiles, geranium, grapefruit, lemon, mandarin, peppermint, rose, rosemary, yarrow

Hangover fennel, juniper, rosemary

Halitosis (bad breath) bergamot, coriander, fennel, lemon, peppermint

Hiccoughs basil, fennel, mandarin

Indigestion and heartburn angelica seed, basil, bergamot, cajeput, cardamom, chamomiles, cinnamon, coriander, fennel, ginger, juniper, lavender, lemon, lemongrass, lime, mandarin, marjoram, melissa, myrrh, neroli (*nervous*), peppermint, rosemary

IBS (irritable bowel syndrome) carrot seed, chamomiles, ginger, myrrh, neroli, patchouli, petitgrain, yarrow

Liver carrot seed, chamomiles, cypress, geranium, grapefruit, lavender, lemon, mandarin, melissa, peppermint, rose, rosemary, yarrow

Loss of appetite angelica seed, bergamot, black pepper, cardamom, chamomiles, cinnamon, fennel, ginger, hyssop, juniper, lime, palmarosa, peppermint, thyme

Nausea and vomiting basil, black pepper, cardamom, chamomiles, cinnamon, coriander, fennel, ginger, lavender, melissa, peppermint

Obesity black pepper, cardamom, cypress, fennel, ginger, grapefruit, juniper, lemon, rosemary

Sluggish digestion black pepper, fennel, ginger, grapefruit, juniper, lemon, peppermint

Spleen chamomiles

Stomach pains chamomiles, fennel, ginger, lavender, marjoram, melissa, peppermint, rosemary

Stomach ulcers chamomiles, lemon, marjoram

Travel sickness ginger, mandarin, peppermint

Worms and intestinal parasites bergamot, chamomiles, eucalyptus, geranium, juniper, lavender, myrrh, rosemary, tea tree, thyme

Genito-urinary system

Childbirth clary sage, jasmine, lavender, neroli, palmarosa

Cystitis angelica seed, bergamot, cajeput, carrot seed, chamomiles, cypress, eucalyptus, frankincense, geranium, juniper, lavender, lemon, myrtle, niaouli, palmarosa, pine, ravensara, sandalwood, tea tree, yarrow

Difficulty in passing urine juniper

Discharges bergamot, cinnamon, lavender, marjoram, myrrh, pine, rose, rosemary, sandalwood, tea tree, thyme

Excessive sexual impulses marjoram

Fluid retention angelica seed, benzoin, carrot seed, cedarwood, chamomiles, cypress, eucalyptus, fennel, geranium, hyssop, juniper, lavender, lemon, lemongrass, pine, rosemary, sandalwood, thyme, yarrow

Frigidity and impotence clary sage, ginger, jasmine, neroli, rose, sandalwood, ylang ylang

Infertility angelica seed, geranium, jasmine, melissa, rose

Insufficiency of milk in nursing mothers fennel, jasmine, lemongrass

Itching (vaginal) bergamot, cedarwood, chamomiles, tea tree

Kidney infections and stones chamomiles, eucalyptus, fennel, geranium, juniper, lemon, sandalwood

Menopause bergamot, carrot seed, chamomiles, clary sage, cypress, fennel, frankincense, geranium, jasmine, lavender, neroli, rose, sandalwood, yarrow, ylang ylang

Menstruation *Heavy blood loss*: chamomiles, cypress, geranium, rose, yarrow; *Irregular*: chamomiles, marjoram, melissa, niaouli, rose, yarrow; *Painful*: angelica seed, cajeput, chamomiles, clary sage, cypress, jasmine, juniper, lavender, marjoram, myrrh, niaouli, peppermint, rose, rosemary, yarrow; *Scanty*: chamomiles, cinnamon, clary sage, fennel, hyssop, juniper, lavender, marjoram, myrrh, niaouli, peppermint, rose, rosemary, thyme, yarrow

Oestrogen (*stimulates body to produce*) fennel

PMS carrot seed, cedarwood, chamomiles, clary sage, cypress, geranium, lavender, marjoram, melissa, neroli, rose, rosemary, sandalwood, ylang ylang

Prostate enlargement jasmine, juniper

Thrush bergamot, eucalyptus, frankincense, lavender, lemon, myrrh, tea tree, thyme

Tonic for the womb clary sage, coriander, jasmine, myrtle, rose

Urinary infections bergamot, cajeput, eucalyptus, juniper, sandalwood, tea tree, thyme

Head disorders

Catarrh basil, black pepper, cajeput, cedarwood, eucalyptus, frankincense, lavender, lemon, lime, myrrh, ravensara, tea tree

Cold sores bergamot, chamomiles, lavender, lemon, melissa, myrrh, tea tree

Earache basil, chamomiles, lavender

Fainting and vertigo basil, black pepper, lavender, peppermint, rosemary

Gum infections (e.g. gingivitis) chamomiles, lemon, myrrh, ravensara, tea tree, thyme

Hair and scalp *Dandruff*: carrot seed, chamomiles, cypress, juniper, lavender, lemon, patchouli, tea tree, thyme; *Dry*: carrot seed, geranium, lavender, palmarosa, rosemary, rosewood, sandalwood; *Lice*: bergamot, eucalyptus, geranium, lavender, lemon, rosemary, tea tree; *Loss of hair*: cedarwood, chamomiles, clary sage, frankincense, geranium, ginger, lavender, rosemary, yarrow; *Oily*: bergamot, cedarwood, clary sage, cypress, frankincense, geranium, lemon, lemongrass, juniper, rosemary, thyme, yarrow; *Sensitive scalp*: chamomiles, lavender

Headaches and migraine basil, chamomiles, lavender, marjoram, peppermint, rosemary

Loss of smell rosemary

Mouth infections and ulcers lemon, myrrh, tea tree, thyme

Nasal polyps basil

Neuralgia basil, black pepper, chamomiles, eucalyptus, geranium, peppermint

Rhinitis and sinusitis basil, cajeput, eucalyptus, lavender, peppermint, ravensara, tea tree, thyme

Toothache cajeput, chamomiles, niaouli, peppermint

Muscular/joint disorders

Aches and pains angelica seed, basil, benzoin, black pepper, cajeput, cardamom, chamomiles, cinnamon, coriander, eucalyptus, frankincense, ginger, juniper, lavender, lemon, lemongrass, lime, marjoram, niaouli, peppermint, pine, ravensara, rosemary, thyme, vetivert, yarrow

Arthritis angelica seed, basil, benzoin, black pepper, cajeput, chamomiles, eucalyptus, ginger, grapefruit, hyssop, juniper, lavender, lemon, marjoram, niaouli, peppermint, pine, rosemary, thyme, vetivert

Bruises black pepper, chamomiles, geranium, hyssop, lavender, marjoram, myrrh, peppermint, rosemary

Cramp basil, black pepper, cardamom, chamomiles, ginger, lavender, marjoram, rosemary, vetivert

Fibrositis benzoin, black pepper, eucalyptus, lavender, peppermint, rosemary

Gout angelica seed, basil, benzoin, cajeput, chamomiles, grapefruit, hyssop, juniper, lemon, lime, rosemary, thyme, yarrow

Inflammation chamomiles, lavender, pine, yarrow

Lack of muscle tone black pepper, lavender, lemongrass, rosemary

Rheumatism angelica seed, basil, black pepper, cajeput, chamomiles, cinnamon, eucalyptus, frankincense, ginger, grapefruit, hyssop, juniper, lavender, lemon, lime, marjoram, myrrh, niaouli, peppermint, pine, rosemary, thyme, vetivert, yarrow

Sprains and strains black pepper, cajeput, chamomiles, eucalyptus, ginger, lavender, lemongrass, marjoram, peppermint, pine, ravensara, rosemary, vetivert, yarrow

Stiffness black pepper, chamomiles, eucalyptus, frankincense, grapefruit, lavender, marjoram, palmarosa, rosemary

---

Nervous system

Alcoholism clary sage, fennel, juniper (*detoxify*), vetivert

Anger chamomiles, cypress, myrtle, neroli, rose, vetivert, yarrow, ylang ylang

Anorexia nervosa basil, benzoin, bergamot, geranium, jasmine, juniper, lavender, mandarin, marjoram, neroli, patchouli, sandalwood, thyme, ylang ylang

Apathy and lethargy ginger, grapefruit, jasmine, lemongrass, lime, mandarin, myrrh, patchouli, rosemary

Change cypress (*enables acceptance*), frankincense (*enables moving on*)

Coldness benzoin, black pepper, frankincense, marjoram, rose

Comfort benzoin, black pepper, cypress, marjoram, rose, rosewood

Confidence (lack of) black pepper, cardamom, coriander, ginger, jasmine

Courage black pepper, coriander, fennel, ginger

Depression basil, bergamot, cardamom, chamomiles, clary sage, geranium, grapefruit, jasmine, lavender, lemongrass, lime, mandarin, melissa, neroli, patchouli, rose, sandalwood, thyme, ylang ylang

Exhaustion angelica seed, benzoin (*mental, emotional, physical*), clary sage (*nervous, physical, sexual*), citronella, coriander, eucalyptus, grapefruit, hyssop, juniper (*emotional and nervous depletion*), lavender, lemon, lime, pine, ravensara, thyme

Fearful clary sage, frankincense, jasmine, lavender, melissa, neroli, sandalwood, ylang ylang

Frigidity and impotence clary sage, ginger, jasmine, neroli, patchouli, peppermint, rose, rosewood, sandalwood, ylang ylang

Grief benzoin, cypress, frankincense, mandarin, marjoram, melissa, neroli, rose

Hysteria and panic chamomiles, clary sage, lavender, marjoram, melissa, neroli

Inability to concentrate basil, cajeput, cardamom, coriander, hyssop, lemon, niaouli, peppermint, ravensara, rosemary

Indecision basil, carrot seed, patchouli

Insomnia chamomiles, lavender, mandarin, marjoram, neroli, rose, sandalwood, ylang ylang

Irritability chamomiles, cypress, lavender, thyme, yarrow

Jealousy rose

Loneliness benzoin, coriander, rose

Memory (poor) basil, black pepper, ginger, hyssop, juniper, rosemary, thyme

Mental fatigue (*clears the mind*) basil, cinnamon, peppermint, rosemary

Mood swings chamomiles, geranium, lavender

Negativity coriander, jasmine, juniper, mandarin, palmarosa, vetivert

Nervous tension basil, cedarwood, clary sage, cypress, geranium, grapefruit, lavender, mandarin, marjoram, neroli, palmarosa, patchouli, petitgrain, rose, sandalwood

Neuralgia basil, black pepper, chamomiles, eucalyptus, geranium, peppermint

Obsessions frankincense, vetivert

Over-sensitivity basil, black pepper, chamomiles, cypress, geranium, lavender

Resentment grapefruit

Sadness benzoin, coriander, jasmine, rose

Sedative bergamot, chamomiles, clary sage, frankincense, marjoram, sandalwood, vetivert

Self-obsession rose

Shock benzoin, mandarin, neroli, peppermint, rose, ylang ylang

---

Respiratory system

Asthma basil, benzoin, cajeput, cypress, eucalyptus, frankincense, hyssop, lavender, lemon, lime, melissa, myrrh, niaouli, peppermint, pine, rosemary, thyme

Breath *Fast*: frankincense, lavender; *Shortness of*: fennel, frankincense, lavender

Bronchitis basil, benzoin, cajeput, cypress, eucalyptus, fennel, frankincense, ginger, hyssop, lavender, lemon, lime, melissa, myrrh, myrtle, niaouli, peppermint, ravensara, rosemary, sandalwood, tea tree, thyme

Catarrh basil, benzoin, black pepper, cajeput, cardamom, cedarwood, eucalyptus, frankincense, ginger, lavender, lemon, myrrh, myrtle, niaouli, ravensara, rosemary, sandalwood, tea tree

Coughs and colds benzoin, bergamot, black pepper, cajeput, cinnamon, coriander, eucalyptus, frankincense, ginger, grapefruit, lavender, lemon, lime, melissa, myrrh, myrtle, niaouli, peppermint, rosemary, rosewood, sandalwood, tea tree, thyme

Cough (whooping) cypress, lavender, rosemary, thyme

Emphysema eucalyptus, frankincense

Flu benzoin, bergamot, black pepper, cinnamon, eucalyptus, fennel, frankincense, ginger, grapefruit, lavender, lemon, lime, myrtle, niaouli, peppermint, rosemary, rosewood, tea tree

Hoarseness and loss of voice myrrh, sandalwood

Laryngitis benzoin, bergamot, cajeput, eucalyptus, lemon, myrrh, niaouli, pine, sandalwood

Sinusitis basil, cajeput, eucalyptus, hyssop, lavender, lemon, myrtle, niaouli, pine, ravensara, tea tree, thyme

Tonsillitis and throat infections benzoin, bergamot, cajeput, eucalyptus, geranium, ginger, hyssop, lavender, lemon, lime, myrrh, niaouli, ravensara, rosewood, sandalwood

Skin

Acne bergamot, carrot seed, cedarwood, chamomiles, cypress, frankincense, grapefruit, juniper, lavender, lemon, lemongrass, lime, mandarin, myrtle, niaouli, palmarosa, patchouli, peppermint, rosemary, sandalwood, tea tree, yarrow, ylang ylang

Ageing skin clary sage, frankincense, lavender, lemon, myrrh, myrtle, neroli, patchouli, rose, rosemary

Allergy chamomiles, lavender, melissa, patchouli, yarrow

Athlete's foot lavender, lemongrass, myrrh, patchouli, tea tree

Bleeding geranium, lemon

Boils and carbuncles bergamot, chamomiles, lavender, lemon, lime, rosemary, tea tree, thyme

Broken capillaries chamomiles, cypress, frankincense, lemon, neroli, rose, sandalwood

Bruises chamomiles, fennel, geranium, hyssop, lavender, marjoram

Burns chamomiles, eucalyptus, lavender, geranium, yarrow

Cellulite angelica seed, cedarwood, cypress, fennel, geranium, grapefruit, juniper, lemon, lime, pine, rosemary, sage

Chapped and cracked skin benzoin, myrrh, palmarosa, patchouli, sandalwood, tea tree

Combination skin geranium, lavender, neroli

Cuts eucalyptus, geranium, lavender, lemon, tea tree

Dermatitis benzoin, juniper, lavender, myrrh, patchouli, peppermint, rosemary

Dry skin benzoin, carrot seed, chamomiles, clary sage, frankincense, geranium, jasmine, lavender, neroli, palmarosa, rose, rosewood, sandalwood, vetivert, ylang ylang

Eczema angelica seed, bergamot, geranium, juniper, lavender, myrrh, palmarosa, patchouli, rosemary, yarrow

Herpes bergamot, eucalyptus, lavender, lemon, lime, melissa, ravensara, tea tree

Inflamed, red, irritated skin benzoin, chamomiles, clary sage, geranium, lavender, myrrh, neroli, patchouli, peppermint, rose

Mature skin carrot seed, clary sage, frankincense, geranium, jasmine, lavender, myrrh, myrtle, neroli, palmarosa, patchouli, rose, rosewood, sandalwood, yarrow

Measles (and other infectious diseases) bergamot, eucalyptus, geranium, lemon, lemongrass, ravensara, rosemary, tea tree

Oily and open pores bergamot, cajeput, cedarwood, citronella, clary sage, cypress, frankincense, geranium, hyssop, juniper, lavender, lemon, lemongrass, lime, mandarin, palmarosa, peppermint, rosewood, sandalwood, tea tree, ylang ylang

Perspiration cypress, lemongrass, tea tree

Psoriasis benzoin, bergamot, cajeput, chamomiles, lavender, niaouli, tea tree, yarrow

Rejuvenate carrot seed, frankincense, lavender, myrrh, myrtle, neroli, rosewood

Scabies lemon, lemongrass, peppermint, rosemary, thyme

Scars carrot seed, jasmine, mandarin, neroli, patchouli

Sensitive chamomiles, geranium, jasmine, lavender, neroli, rose

Sunburn clary sage, lavender, peppermint

Ulcers frankincense, geranium, juniper, lavender, myrrh, tea tree

Varicose veins cypress, geranium, ginger, lemon, neroli, tea tree, yarrow

Warts and verrucae lemon, lime, tea tree

Wounds and sores benzoin, frankincense, geranium, juniper, myrrh, patchouli, tea tree, thyme

Wrinkles carrot seed, clary sage, frankincense, myrrh, palmarosa, patchouli, rose, rosemary, rosewood

Taking it further

Supplies

Denise Brown Essential Oils
Kingshott Business Centre, Hinton Road
Bournemouth BH1 2EF
Tel: +44 (0)1202 708887
www.denisebrown.co.uk

A wide selection of high-quality, pure unadulterated essential oils, base oils, creams and lotions, Bach Flower Remedies, relaxation music, etc. are available from Denise Brown.

Aromatherapy training

BEAUMONT COLLEGE OF NATURAL MEDICINE

Wells, Somerset
Tel: +44 (0)1749 675090
www.beaumontcollege.co.uk

Training courses under the direction of Denise Whichello Brown.

AROMATHERAPY COUNCIL

www.aromatherapycouncil.co.uk

Training advice and tips for choosing an aromatherapy training course.

INTERNATIONAL FEDERATION OF PROFESSIONAL AROMATHERAPISTS (IFPA)

Tel: +44 (0)1455 637987
www.ifparoma.org

Accredited courses and practitioners.

INTERNATIONAL FEDERATION OF AROMATHERAPISTS (IFA)

Tel: +44 (0)20 8992 9605
www.ifaroma.org

Accredited courses and practitioners.

International Therapy Examination Council (ITEC)

Tel: +44 (0)20 8994 4141
www.itecworld.co.uk

Accredited courses.

GENERAL REGULATORY COUNCIL FOR COMPLEMENTARY THERAPIES

Tel: +44 (0)870 3144031
www.grcct.org

The UK Federal Regulator for Complementary Therapies.

AROMATHERAPY ON-LINE CORRESPONDENCE COURSE

www.beaumontcollege.co.uk/correspond.html

A free interactive internet aromatherapy e-course for use on friends and family.

The publisher has used its best endeavours to ensure that the URLs for external websites referred to in this book are correct and active at the time of going to press. However, the publisher has no responsibility for the websites and can make no guarantee that a site will remain live or that the content is or will remain appropriate.

Further reading

To complement the information in this book why not read Denise Whichello Brown's other books in this series:

Get Started in Massage
Teach Yourself Detox
Teach Yourself Indian Head Massage
Teach Yourself Hand Reflexology
Your Evening Class – Complementary Therapies
Available from most literary outlets

Test your knowledge answers

Chapter 1

1 *a Hippocrates is the 'Father of Medicine'*
2 *Kyphi was a famous perfume and incense*
3 *Ayurvedic medicine originates in India*
4 *b Avicenna invented distillation*
5 *Herbs were used during the plagues as protection*
6 *b Gattefossé coined the word 'aromatherapy'*

Chapter 2

1 *Distillation is the most widely used method of extraction*
2 *Expression is used for citrus oils*
3 *Solvent extraction produces an absolute*
4 *Resinoids are employed as fixatives to prolong the fragrance of an oil*
5 *Enfleurage is too time-consuming and labour intensive*

Chapter 3

1 *Essential oils should be stored in amber bottles*
2 *Essential oils vary greatly in price*
3 *a bath/shower – six drops. b footbath/hand bath – six drops. c compress – six drops. d gargle – two drops.*
4 *Three drops of essential oil are blended with 10 ml of carrier oil*

Chapter 4

1 *Mineral oil clogs the pores and does not have the nutritional constituents of vegetable oils*
2 *Quality, texture, absorbability and aroma*
3 *a, b, d Sweet almond, apricot kernel and grapeseed are often used on their own*
4 *Evening primrose oil is often taken in capsule form*
5 *c Wheatgerm oil contains high levels of vitamin E*

Chapter 5

1 *b basil*
2 *d chamomile*
3 *a citronella*
4 *d ginger*
5 *d lavender*
6 *e myrrh*
7 *a myrtle*
8 *a peppermint*
9 *d tea tree*
10 *d ylang ylang*

Chapter 6

1 *38*
2 *Mimulus*
3 *Impatiens*
4 *Olive*
5 *Walnut*
6 *Crab Apple*
7 *Honeysuckle*
8 *Larch*

Chapter 7

1 *Keep all areas covered, other than the part you are treating*
2 *White is the best colour to wear when giving a massage*
3 *Place one pillow under the head and one under the knees*
4 *No, you should never massage with undiluted oils*
5 *Friction loosens knots and nodules*
6 *Pressure is on the way up the legs*
7 *The abdomen is massaged in a clockwise direction*
8 *Choose any three of the following: relaxing, relieves skin problems, headaches, nasal problems, slows the ageing process, increases clarity of thought*

Chapter 8

1 *At least six to eight glasses of water should be drunk daily*
2 *Sugar is linked with heart disease, obesity, mood changes and tooth decay (choose two)*
3 *Snack, salads, stir-fry, sandwiches, soups, casseroles, omelettes (choose two)*
4 *The Western diet is usually more acid*
5 *Use organically grown unsprayed produce for juicing*

Chapter 9

1 *Iron tablets are given in cases of anaemia*
2 *You would put six drops in the bath*
3 *Olive is indicated for exhaustion*
4 *To sweeten the breath chew parsley*
5 *In 20 ml of carrier oil blend three drops of frankincense and three drops of lavender*

6   *b To help low blood pressure use three drops of thyme/three drops of rosemary*
7   *Add six drops ginger to a footbath or hand bath*
8   *a To improve varicose veins use cypress, lemon and geranium*

Chapter 10

1   *Aromatherapy is particularly useful for the psychological state of an anorexic*
2   *a Use jasmine/rose to help depression and raise self-esteem*
3   *For vaginal thrush use myrrh/tea tree*
4   *Sugar should be eliminated from the diet of a person in cases of candida*
5   *a For constipation choose fennel/juniper/marjoram*
6   *For indigestion squeeze half a lemon into a glass of water*
7   *Fennel is useful for weight loss and detoxification*
8   *Crab Apple is indicated for cleansing*

Chapter 11

1   *a For pain relief in cases of osteoarthritis choose black pepper/ ginger*
2   *To encourage detoxification use cypress/fennel*
3   *To curb inflammation choose chamomile/yarrow*
4   *The big toe is commonly affected by gout*
5   *No, it is contraindicated to massage an inflamed joint*

Chapter 12

1   *The sebaceous glands are underactive in cases of dry skin*
2   *Use nine drops of essential oil to a 30 ml facial blend*
3   *For dry skin choose carrot seed, rose and sandalwood*

4 *Cosmetics containing alcohol strip moisture from the surface of the skin*
5 *The sebaceous glands are producing too much sebum in cases of oily skin*
6 *Oily skin is most common during puberty*
7 *For oily skin choose bergamot and lemon*
8 *For rejuvenation and ageing skin choose rose and frankincense*
9 *Lavender and tea tree may be applied to individual spots*
10 *Essential oils:*
    a *Chamomile – blonde hair*
    b *Carrot seed – ginger hair*
    c *Rosemary/rosewood – dark hair*

Chapter 13

1 *To relieve menstrual pain choose lavender and peppermint*
2 *To relieve hot flushes choose cypress and peppermint*
3 *Walnut helps a woman to cope with the change*
4 *To reduce the cravings for sweet things try fennel*
5 *To balance mood swings try chamomile and geranium*
6 *Impatiens is indicated for irritability and impatience*

Chapter 14

1 *Ginger and mandarin can help combat morning sickness*
2 *Inhale the oils from a tissue or add them to a morning bath to combat morning sickness*
3 *Three oils which can help to prevent stretchmarks are frankincense, neroli and rose*
4 *b Clary sage/lavender/rose would be suitable for childbirth*
5 *To treat mastitis use the compress method*
6 *For a baby up to 12 months use one drop of essential oil in the bath*

7   *a Chamomile is useful for colic*
8   *For a child aged 1–5 use two drops in the bath*
9   *Choose lavender and myrtle to treat a child's cough*
10 *Lavender would help to heal a cut*

Chapter 15

1   *Add two drops of essential oil to the final rinse when washing by hand*
2   *Sprinkle six drops of essential oil on to squares of blotting paper*
3   *Jasmine and rose are particularly suitable for sexual arousal in a woman*
4   *b To treat impotence you would use black pepper/ginger/jasmine*
5   *Larch boosts confidence*

Index

Image credits

Front cover: © David Cook/blueshiftstudios/Alamy

Back cover: © Jakub Semeniuk/iStockphoto.com, © Royalty-Free/ Corbis, © agencyby/iStockphoto.com, © Andy Cook/ iStockphoto.com, © Christopher Ewing/iStockphoto.com, © zebicho – Fotolia.com, © Geoffrey Holman/iStockphoto.com, © Photodisc/Getty Images, © James C. Pruitt/iStockphoto.com, © Mohamed Saber – Fotolia.com

Lightning Source UK Ltd.
Milton Keynes UK
UKOW05f2325171016

285528UK00018B/460/P